Current Concepts in Arrhythmogenic Cardiomyopathy

Second Edition

ONLINE ACCESS

The purchase of a new copy of this book entitles the first retail purchaser to free personal online access to a digital version of this edition.

Please send a copy of your purchase receipt to info@cardiotext.com with subject ARVC2 EBOOK, and we will email you a redemption code along with instructions on how to access the digital file.

Current Concepts in Arrhythmogenic Cardiomyopathy

Second Edition

Editors:

Prof. Dr. CORINNA BRUNCKHORST
Co-Director, Cardiac Arrhythmia Service
University Heart Center, Zurich, Switzerland

PD Dr. ARDAN M. SAGUNER
Senior Consultant, Cardiac Arrhythmia Service
University Heart Center, Zurich, Switzerland

Prof. Dr. FIRAT DURU
Director, Cardiac Arrhythmia Service
University Heart Center, Zurich, Switzerland

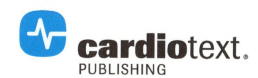

Second Edition

First Edition © 2014 Corinna Brunckhorst, Firat Duru

Second Edition © 2021 Corinna Brunckhorst, Ardan M. Saguner, Firat Duru

The first edition of this book is entitled Current Concepts in Arrhythmogenic Right Ventricular Cardiomyopathy/Dysplasia.

Cardiotext Publishing, LLC
3405 W. 44th Street
Minneapolis, Minnesota 55410
USA
www.cardiotextpublishing.com

Any updates to this book may be found at: www.cardiotextpublishing.com/ electrophysiology-heart-rhythm-mgmt/current-con-cepts-in-arrhythmogenic-cardiomyopathy-second-edition

Comments, inquiries, and requests for bulk sales can be directed to the publisher at: info@cardiotextpublishing.com.

Unless otherwise stated, all figures and tables in this book and on the cover are used courtesy of the authors.

The pathology image on the front cover is provided courtesy of Dr. Peter Bode from the University Hospital Zurich.

Library of Congress Control Number: 2020922050

ISBN: 978-1-942909-50-7
eISBN: 978-1-942909-51-4

Printed in the United States

1 2 3 4 5 6 7   25 24 23 22 21

Dedication

We sincerely thank all patients with arrhythmogenic cardiomyopathy who agreed to be enrolled in clinical research studies and have helped to substantially advance our understanding of this challenging disease. It is a tremendous privilege to interact with our collaborators and friends around the globe in an attempt to advance this field to new frontiers. Furthermore, we are immensely thankful for the invaluable endorsement of our sponsors, as it is only due to their enormous generosity that our work is rendered possible. In addition, we are greatly indebted to our exceptional mentors, who have paved the way for us to follow their paths.

We are more than grateful for the affection and support of our families who help us maintain our rhythm. Ultimately, this book is dedicated, in love and gratitude, to the memory of our dear parents Sieglinde Brunckhorst, Oylar Saguner, and Nurettin Duru. They will always remain in our hearts.

Table of Contents

Contributors

Editors

CORINNA BRUNCKHORST, MD
Co-Director, Cardiac Arrhythmia Service, University Heart Center, Zurich, Switzerland

ARDAN M. SAGUNER, MD
Senior Consultant, Cardiac Arrhythmia Service, University Heart Center, Zurich, Switzerland

FIRAT DURU, MD
Director, Cardiac Arrhythmia Service, University Heart Center, Zurich, Switzerland

Contributors

Deniz Akdis, MD
Cardiology Resident/ARVC Fellow, Cardiac Arrhythmia Service, University Heart Center, Zurich, Switzerland

Areej Aljehani, MSc
Institute of Cardiovascular Sciences, University of Birmingham, Department of Cardiology, University Hospital Birmingham, Birmingham, UK

Angeliki Asimaki, PhD
St. George's, University of London, London, UK

Fabrizio R. Assis, MD
ARVC Program, Division of Cardiology, Johns Hopkins University School of Medicine, Baltimore, Maryland, USA

Cristina Basso, MD, PhD
Department of Cardiac, Thoracic and Vascular Sciences and Public Health, University of Padua Medical School, Padua, Italy

Maria A. Baturova, MD, PhD
Department of Cardiology, Lund University, Lund, Sweden; Research Park, Saint Petersburg State University, Saint Petersburg, Russia

Laurens P. Bosman, MD
Department of Cardiology, University Medical Center, University of Utrecht; Netherlands Heart Institute, Utrecht, The Netherlands

Mimount Bourfiss, MD
Department of Cardiology, University Medical Center Utrecht, Utrecht, The Netherlands

Carlos Bueno-Beti, PhD
St. George's, University of London, London, UK

Julia Cadrin-Tourigny, MD
Department of Medicine and Cardiovascular Genetics Center, Montreal Heart Institute, Université de Montréal, Montréal, Canada; Johns Hopkins ARVC Program, Johns Hopkins Division of Cardiology, Department of Medicine, Johns Hopkins University, Baltimore, Maryland, USA

Hugh Calkins, MD
Division of Cardiology, Johns Hopkins Medical Institutions, Baltimore, Maryland, USA

Marina Cerrone, MD
Inherited Arrhythmias Clinic, Heart Rhythm Center, Leon H. Charney Division of Cardiology, New York University School of Medicine, New York, New York, USA

Shing Fai Chan, PhD
Krannert Institute of Cardiology, Indiana
University, Indianapolis, Indiana, USA

Stephen P. Chelko, PhD
Department of Biomedical Sciences, Florida
State University College of Medicine,
Tallahassee, Florida, USA

Huei-sheng Vincent Chen, MD, PhD
Krannert Institute of Cardiology, Indiana
University, Indianapolis, Indiana, USA

Liang Chen, MD, PhD
State Key Laboratory of Cardiovascular
Disease, Fuwai Hospital; National Center for
Cardiovascular Diseases, Chinese Academy of
Medical Sciences (CAMS) and Peking Union
Medical College (PUMC), Beijing, P. R. China

Monica De Gaspari, MD
Department of Cardiac, Thoracic and Vascular
Sciences and Public Health, University of Padua
Medical School, Padua, Italy

Mario Delmar, MD, PhD
Leon H. Charney Division of Cardiology, New
York University School of Medicine, New York,
New York, USA

Larissa Fabritz, MD
Institute of Cardiovascular Sciences, University
of Birmingham; Department of Cardiology,
University Hospital Birmingham,
Birmingham, UK

Jodie Ingles, GradDipGenCouns, PhD, MPH
Agnes Ginges Centre for Molecular Cardiology,
Centenary Institute, Sydney;
Sydney Medical School, Faculty of Medicine
and Health, University of Sydney;
Department of Cardiology, Royal Prince Alfred
Hospital, Sydney, Australia

Robert M. Hamilton, MD, MHSc, FRCP(C)
The Labatt Family Heart Centre and Division
of Cardiology Department of Pediatrics, and
Translational Medicine Program, The Hospital
for Sick Children and University of Toronto,
Toronto, Ontario, Canada

Richard Hauer, MD, PhD
Department of Cardiology, University Medical
Center Utrecht; Netherlands Heart Institute,
Utrecht, The Netherlands

Cynthia A. James, PhD, ScM
Johns Hopkins ARVC Program, Johns Hopkins
Division of Cardiology, Department of
Medicine, Johns Hopkins University, Baltimore,
Maryland, USA

Daniel P. Judge, MD
Medical University of South Carolina;
Fellowship Program Director, Cardiology;
Director of Cardiovascular Genetics,
Section of Advanced Heart Failure &
Transplant, Charleston, South Carolina, USA

Manish Kalla, MD
Department of Cardiology, University Hospital
Birmingham, Institute of Cardiovascular
Sciences, University of Birmingham,
Birmingham, UK

Justin Lowenthal, BS
Department of Biomedical Engineering,
Johns Hopkins School of Medicine, Baltimore,
Maryland, USA

Frank I. Marcus, MD
Professor Emeritus, Department of Cardiology,
Sarver Heart Center, University of Arizona
Health Science Center, Tucson, Arizona, USA

Pyotr G. Platonov, MD, PhD
Department of Cardiology, Lund University,
Lund, Sweden

Alexandros Protonotarios, MD
Institute of Cardiovascular Science, University
College London, London, UK

Stefania Rizzo, MD, PhD
Department of Cardiac, Thoracic and Vascular
Sciences and Public Health, University of Padua
Medical School, Padua, Italy

Jeffrey E. Saffitz, MD, PhD
Department of Pathology, Beth Israel Deaconess
Medical Center, Boston, Massachusetts, USA

Christopher Semsarian, MBBS, PhD, MPH
Agnes Ginges Centre for Molecular Cardiology,
Centenary Institute, Sydney;
Sydney Medical School, Faculty of Medicine
and Health, University of Sydney;
Department of Cardiology, Royal Prince Alfred
Hospital, Sydney, Australia

Laura Sommerfeld, MSc
Institute of Cardiovascular Sciences, University
of Birmingham, Birmingham, UK

Jiangping Song, MD, PhD
State Key Laboratory of Cardiovascular
Disease, Fuwai Hospital; National Center for
Cardiovascular Diseases, Chinese Academy of
Medical Sciences (CAMS) and Peking Union
Medical College (PUMC), Beijing, P. R. China

Harikrishna Tandri, MD
ARVC Program, Division of Cardiology,
Johns Hopkins University School of Medicine,
Baltimore, Maryland, USA

Anneline S. J. M. te Riele, MD, PhD
Department of Cardiology, University Medical
Center, University of Utrecht; Netherlands
Heart Institute, Utrecht, The Netherlands

Gaetano Thiene, MD
Department of Cardiac, Thoracic and Vascular
Sciences and Public Health, University of Padua
Medical School, Padua, Italy

Adalena Tsatsopoulou, MD
Naxos General Hospital, Naxos, Greece

Leslie Tung, PhD
Department of Biomedical Engineering,
Johns Hopkins School of Medicine, Baltimore,
Maryland, USA

Chantal J. M. van Opbergen, PhD
Leon H. Charney Division of Cardiology, New
York University School of Medicine, New York,
New York, USA

J. Peter van Tintelen, MD, PhD
Department of Medical Genetics, University
Medical Center Utrecht, University of Utrecht,
Utrecht, The Netherlands

Chuan-yu Wei, PhD
Krannert Institute of Cardiology, Indiana
University, Indianapolis, Indiana, USA

Preface

Arrhythmogenic cardiomyopathy continues to be a challenging clinical entity, for which the diagnosis, risk stratification, and therapy have evolved over the last three decades. When we published the first edition of this book in 2014, our primary focus was on arrhythmogenic right ventricular cardiomyopathy (ARVC), which is the most common and typical form of arrhythmogenic cardiomyopathy. In recent years, there has been mounting evidence that the disease is not confined to the right ventricle, but in most cases, it involves both ventricles. Therefore, we have adapted the title of this edition to be *Current Concepts in Arrhythmogenic Cardiomyopathy, Second Edition.*

All cardiomyopathies can predispose the affected patients to the occurrence of ventricular arrhythmias. The main difference between arrhythmogenic cardiomyopathy and other forms of cardiomyopathies is that, in the former, life-threatening arrhythmias may occur early and out of proportion to the degree of the underlying myocardial substrate. This poses the patients who are typically young and athletic at high risk for sudden cardiac death. When we established the Zurich ARVC Program in 2011, our primary aim was to increase awareness for this challenging disease. Our program, which was initially supported by the Georg and Bertha Schwyzer-Winiker Foundation, has received other generous support and research funds from the Baugarten Foundation, Dr. Hans-Peter Wild / USZ Foundation, Swiss Heart Foundation, and Swiss National Science Foundation (SNF). Therefore, we were fortunate to focus our efforts on providing clinical excellence for the care of these patients and promoting in-depth basic and clinical research for this disease. Moreover, in the course of this decade, we were able to organize four international symposia to create a platform for exchange of knowledge and initiate global collaboration by convening key opinion leaders for arrhythmogenic cardiomyopathy from around the world in Zurich.

Current Concepts in Arrhythmogenic Cardiomyopathy, Second Edition includes 16 chapters on various basic and clinical science aspects of arrhythmogenic cardiomyopathy. It includes a broad spectrum of topics, including pathophysiology, molecular mechanisms, and genetic background of disease, as well as its clinical presentation, diagnosis, risk stratification, and therapy. Our ultimate goal is to offer a useful guide to help medical caregivers provide the best possible care for their patients and update them with state-of-the-art knowledge on this disease. We sincerely hope that *Current Concepts in Arrhythmogenic Cardiomyopathy, Second Edition* fulfills this purpose.

We wish to thank all the contributing authors for their invaluable collaborations and for being part of this project.

—*The Editors*

Abbreviations

ACE	angiotensin-converting enzyme		LGE	late gadolinium enhancement
ACM	arrhythmogenic cardiomyopathy		LV	left ventricle; left ventricular
AF	atrial fibrillation		LVEF	left ventricular ejection fraction
ALVC	arrhythmogenic left ventricular cardiomyopathy		MACE	major adverse cardiovascular events
APC	adenomatous polyposis coli		MCFA	medium-chain fatty acids
ARVC	arrhythmogenic right ventricular cardiomyopathy		MMP	matrix metalloproteinase
			MRI	magnetic resonance imaging
AV	atrioventricular		NCAD	N-cadherin
β-OHB	β-hydroxybutyrate		NFκB	nuclear factor κB
BCDS	bilateral cardiac sympathetic denervation		NGS	next-generation sequencing
			NIPS	noninvasive programmed stimulation
BrS	Brugada syndrome		NLVS	nonischemic left ventricular scar
CAAR	chimeric autoantibody receptor		NRVMs	neonatal rat ventricular myocytes
CMR	cardiac magnetic resonance		NSVT	nonsustained ventricular tachycardia
CMs	cardiomyocytes		Nt-BNP	N-terminal pro-brain natriuretic peptide
CPVT	catecholaminergic polymorphic ventricular tachycardia		PKC	protein kinase C
Cx43	connexin43		PKP2	plakophilin-2
DCM	dilated cardiomyopathy		PLN	phospholamban
DPI	days postinjection		PPAR	peroxisome proliferator-activated receptor
DSC2	desmocollin-2			
DSG2	desmoglein-2		PTF-V1	P-terminal negative force in lead V1
DSP	desmoplakin		PVC	premature ventricular contraction
EC4	extracellular cadherin 4		RAAS	renin-angiotensin-aldosterone system
EC5/EA	extracellular cadherin 5/extracellular articulating		ROS	reactive oxygen species
			RV	right ventricular
ECG	electrocardiogram		RyR	ryanodine receptors
ELISA	enzyme-linked immunosorbent assay		SAECGs	signal-averaged electrocardiograms
EP	electrophysiology		SAP97	synapse-associated protein 97
FAO	fatty acid oxidation		SCD	sudden cardiac death
HCM	hypertrophic cardiomyopathy		shRNA	short hairpin RNA
HTx	heart transplant/heart transplantation		TAD	terminal activation duration/delay
ICD	implantable cardioverter-defibrillator		TFC	Task Force Criteria
iPSC	induced pluripotent stem cells		TTE	transthoracic echocardiography
iPSC-CMs	induced pluripotent stem cell-derived cardiomyocytes		VA	ventricular arrhythmia
			VF	ventricular fibrillation
JUP	plakoglobin		VT	ventricular tachycardia
KO	knockout		WES	whole exome sequencing
LCFA	long-chain fatty acids		WT	wildtype

Introduction

Right ventricular cardiomyopathy/dysplasia (ARVC/D) is considered to be a newly identified, rare disease. However, it is neither. It has been a well-recognized entity since the publication of 24 cases in 1982.[1] Subsequently, there have been a plethora of articles describing the various aspects of ARVC/D including ECG characteristics, frequent involvement of the left ventricle, and recognition of familial inheritance. It is now recognized that it is not rare, as shown by a recent report of 1001 patients and family members with this disease.[2]

ARVC/D was recognized several hundred years ago, as documented by Gaetano Thiene.[3] He noted that the first report of ARVC/D was published by Lancisi in 1736.[4] The first detailed pathological description was published by Laennec in 1819.[5] There followed a lack of reports of ARVC/D until 1961 when Dalla Volta et al. published observations of patients with "auricular-ization of the right ventricle."[6] Dalla Volta emphasized the hemodynamic dysfunction of the right ventricle. Recognition of the disease as a distinct entity was made by Guy Fontaine in the 1970s from patients who were referred for treatment of ventricular tachycardia but did not have ischemic heart disease or congestive heart failure.[7] The ventricular tachycardia was initiated from the right ventricle with a left bundle branch block morphology. There were 24 patients with similar morphologies in their ECGs during ventricular tachycardia, and these patients had similar diagnostic criteria that was described as a syndrome and published by Marcus et al. in 1982.[1] A familial inheritance was also observed. Once these observations were published, the disease became well recognized as a frequent cause of ventricular tachycardia and became a disease entity.

What does this sequence of the discovery of ARVC/D indicate? How many disease entities are still undiscovered? The answer to this question is unknown, but the sequence of the recognition of the discovery of ARVC/D indicates that there may be a number of diseases that are yet to be uncovered. The availability of genetics should assist in the discovery of new diseases.

—*Frank Marcus, MD*

References

1. Marcus FI, Fontaine GH, Guiraudon G, et al. Right ventricular dysplasia: A report of 24 cases. Circulation. 1982;65:384–398.

2. Groeneweg JA, Bhonsale A, James CA, et al. Clinical presentation, long term follow-up, and outcomes of 1001 arrhythmogenic right ventricular dysplasia/cardiomyopathy patients and family members. *Circ Cardiovascular Genet.* 2015;8:437–446.

3. Thiene G. The research venture in arrhythmogenic right ventricular cardiomyopathy: A paradigm of translational medicine. *Eur Heart J.* 2015;36:837–846.

4. Lancisi GM. De motu cardis et aneuysmatibus. Caput V. Naples: excedebat. Felix-Carolus Musca, 1936.

5. Laennec RTH. De l'ausutation mediate au trané du diagnostic des maladies des poumons et du Coeur. Paris: Brosson & Chaudé, 1819.

6. Dalla Volta S, Farneli O, Maschio G. Le syndrome clinique et hemodynamique de l'auricularisation du ventricule droit. *Arch Mal Coeur.* 1965;58:1129–1143.

7. Fontaine G, Frank R, Vedel J, Grosgogeat Y, Carbrol C, Facquet J. Stimulation studies and epicardial mapping in ventricular tachycardia: study of mechanisms and selection for surgery. In: Kulbertus HE (ed). *Reentrant Arrhythmias.* Lancaster, PA: MTPP Publishing, 1977:334–350.

The History of Naxos Disease: Landmarks in the History of the Disorder

Alexandros Protonotarios, MD; Adalena Tsatsopoulou, MD

> *"The whole art of medicine is in observation."*
>
> –William Osler
> "The Hospital as a College," *Aequanimitas*

Clinical Observations

In the winter of 1984, in a mountain village of Naxos, a 24-year-old male presented to the rural surgery with an episode of sustained ventricular tachycardia (VT). His previous history of arrhythmia had started 7 years ago with syncope followed by a burst of episodes of VT. Following the diagnosis of Ebstein's anomaly, the patient had undergone a tricuspid valve replacement in an Athens hospital. Since then, he suffered one or two episodes of sustained VT each year, presenting with vomiting; the episodes were well tolerated, and he was defibrillated to restore the sinus rhythm on all occasions. Interestingly, this young man had severe hyperkeratotic lesions on his palms and soles, causing him suffering as he worked in his agricultural activities, and extremely woolly hair unlike his other family members. The patient's electrocardiogram (ECG) was quite abnormal with low voltages, precordial QRS prolongation, and repolarization abnormalities, while his chest x-ray showed huge cardiomegaly attributed to extreme right ventricular outflow tract (RVOT) dilatation. That episode of sustained VT was as the previous ones: unresponsive to medical treatment and terminated by defibrillation in an Athens tertiary hospital, where the patient was transported by a helicopter.

Naxos, the biggest of the Cyclades islands in Greece, is located at the middle of the Aegean Sea and has 20,000 inhabitants. In the early 1980s, the only connection from Naxos to Athens was an 8- to 10-hour trip by boat to the Athenian port of Piraeus, scheduled every other day. There was neither a hospital nor a primary health center on the island. A pair of young, married doctors, Nikos Protonotarios and Adalena Tsatsopoulou, had chosen Naxos, as Nikos' homeland, to serve their obligatory rural service in order to achieve a license to practice. On that case, their first impression was that an association of severe ventricular arrhythmias (VAs) with palmoplantar keratoderma in a young person was likely a syndromic defect, since two rare phenotypes coexisted.[1] Nevertheless, such an association did not exist in their medical textbooks at the time. A few months later, during a social event, they were extremely surprised to meet a 32-year-old professional photographer with the same hair and cutaneous features, who discussed with them his problem of chest discomfort and recurrent VA episodes; after extensive evaluation, he had already been given a diagnosis of dilated cardiomyopathy (DCM). The patient's ECG showed intraventricular conduction delay and precordial repolarization changes.

Later in the same year, a 17-year-old girl from a different village on the island died suddenly while at school. She had the same cutaneous phenotype as the two other patients. Interestingly, a couple of years previously, she had been diagnosed with DCM after an episode of syncope (**Figure 1.1**). The incidence of three young patients presenting an extremely rare skin condition also associated with rare events of severe VAs or sudden death and belonging to a population pool of around 4,000 (all residents of villages occupying the moun-

tainous region of Naxos) warranted further investigation. The three patients were apparently not related. However, the two doctors suspected familial occurrence of the defects, so they decided to visit the family of the girl. There were two older siblings with woolly hair and palmoplantar keratoderma. The eldest brother at 26 years old had already suffered episodes of syncope and, after complete physical examination, 12-lead resting ECG, and chest x-ray, could be suspected of having DCM (**Figure 1.2**). The younger brother, who was 17 years old, was asymptomatic but had abnormal ECG findings (**Figure 1.3**).

On a warm, sunny day by the seashore, Drs Protonotarios and Tsatsopoulou noticed a well-developed young boy with woolly hair enjoying the sea. On a closer look, keratoses on palms and soles were obvious. Carefully approaching the family, they were given permission to do an evaluation of the boy, and the 12-lead resting ECG was consistent with a myocardial defect (**Figure 1.4**). The increasing data of a syndromic potentially lethal cardiac disorder running in those families challenged the physicians to make a thorough investigation of other families with this cutaneous condition. This study was ultimately designed and performed

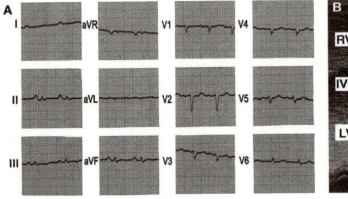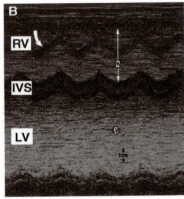

FIGURE 1.1 Resting 12-lead ECG (**A**) and M-mode echocardiography (**B**) of the 17-year-old girl as were recorded in a clinic visit prior to her suffering sudden cardiac death (SCD), are presented. Right and left ventricular dilatation and hypokinesia as well as paradoxical interventricular septal motion are observed. An echodense muscular type band (**white arrow**) is obvious in the right ventricle. Abbreviations: IVS, interventricular septum; LV, left ventricle; RV, right ventricle. (Figure reproduced from Protonotarios et al., *Cardiovasc Pathol.* 2014;13(4),185–194.[1])

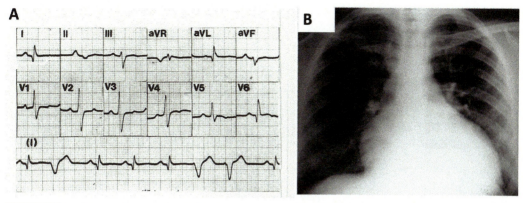

FIGURE 1.2 Recording from baseline 12-lead ECG (**A**) and chest x-ray (**B**) in a 26-year-old man with Naxos disease and severe biventricular involvement are presented. (Figure reproduced from Protonotarios et al., *Cardiovasc Pathol.* 2014;13(4),185–194.[1])

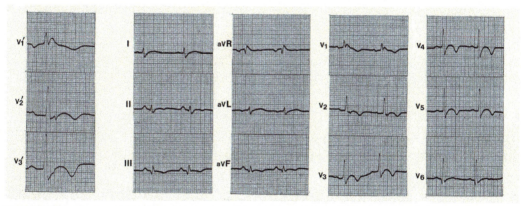

FIGURE 1.3 Resting 12-lead ECG of the asymptomatic 17-year-old man showing QRS of right bundle branch block morphology with inferior and extensive precordial T-wave inversions is presented. Right-sided precordial leads are also presented (V1', V2', V3').

on the whole island by Drs. Protonotarios and Tsatsopoulou. The investigation went on to reveal more families living in Naxos, as well as others in Athens but of Naxian origin, with the affected persons being closely related. An autosomal recessive, inherited disorder could be postulated. All but one young boy, age 6, presented similar cardiac findings.

Description of a New Syndrome

In those pre-internet times, researching the scientific literature in Greece was only available by looking up studies in the printed *Index Medicus* volumes in Athens. Therefore, after

persistent and continuous searching for a whole month into myriad lemmas embedded into thin and densely written pages, the two doctors were convinced that the observed syndromic association had not been described in any publications since 1895.

The permission Dr. Protonotarios gained by the 401 Army Hospital to perform echocardiographic evaluations for all of the patients himself was critical to the whole investigation. Impressed by the kinetic abnormalities of the RV (**Figure 1.5**), he focused on a detailed evaluation of RV structure and function and performed the echocardiographic evaluation and follow-up in all patients himself, following standard protocols.[2] The common find-

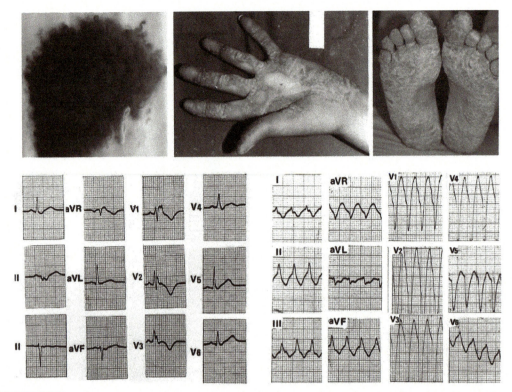

FIGURE 1.4 Representative photographs demonstrating the woolly hair and palmoplantar keratoderma (**top**). Resting 12-lead ECG is shown in **bottom left** and an episode of sustained VT in **bottom right**.

ings of RVOT dilatation and localized kinetic abnormalities of the RV free wall together with the precordial repolarization changes led the doctors to notice in the *Index Medicus* a publication in *Circulation* by Frank Marcus and Guy Fontaine from 2 years earlier.[3] Eventually, the condition called "arrhythmogenic RV dysplasia" (now referred to as arrhythmogenic RV cardiomyopathy or ARVC) was the closest description to the cardiomyopathy their patients presented with. The first observations in 9 patients belonging to 4 families were submitted to the *British Heart Journal* in February 1986 and published without any revision just 4 months later.[4] Alongside the initial report in *Circulation* in 1982, it was one of the first descriptions of ARVC patients. Notably, both left ventricular (LV) involvement and atrial fibrillation (AF) were described in these patients, features that were not linked to ARVC until much later on.

Following the breakthrough publication in *The New England Journal of Medicine* by the Padua group,[5] the 2 doctors sent a letter to the editor of the *NEJM* stressing the presentation of a broad clinical spectrum of ARVC in the Naxos series and an observation of inflammatory findings in myocardial specimens.[6] They also postulated a potential relationship between Veneto and Naxos patients, due to the long-standing occupation of Naxos island after the 13th century. That letter would initiate the link between their research and the ARVC community of London and Padua later on.

Within 4 years, 14 more patients of Naxian origin situated in Athens and Frankfurt who had the combination of palmoplantar keratosis, woolly hair, and ARVC had been identified. They were fully investigated and put in a standard prospective follow-up protocol designed by the two doctors. Heart biopsy specimens were consistent with ARVC (**Figure 1.6**). Electro-

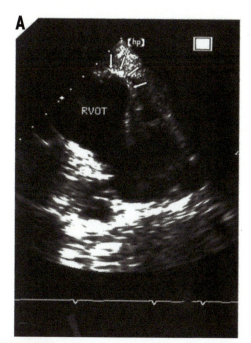
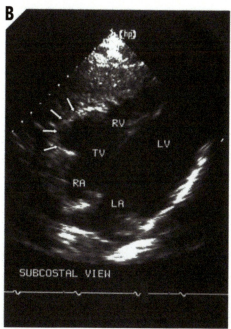

FIGURE 1.5   Two-dimensional echocardiographic images recorded from a patient with Naxos disease (**Panel A**). An aneurysm of the RV outflow tract (**white arrows**) is exhibited by a modified parasternal long-axis view (**Panel B**). An aneurysm of posterior wall of the RV just below the tricuspid valve (**white arrows**) is exhibited by a subcostal four-chamber view. Abbreviations: LA, left atrium; LV, left ventricle; RA, right atrium; RV, right ventricle; RVOT, right ventricular outflow tract; TV, tricuspid valve. (Figure reproduced from Protonotarios et al., *J Am Coll Cardiol.* 2001;38:1477–1484.[2])

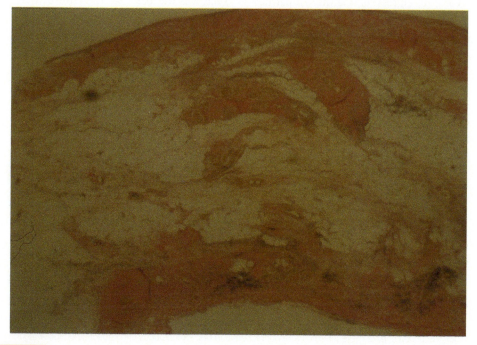

FIGURE 1.6   Hematoxylin-eosin stained section of the anterior wall of the RV shows fibrofatty replacement of cardiac myocytes in the mediomural layers. (Figure reproduced from McKoy et al., *Lancet.* 2000;355:2119–2124.[10])

physiological investigations had been performed in Guy's Hospital, London and in Jean Rostand Hospital, Paris by Dr. Guy Fontaine.

It is a universal truth that life is mostly unexpectable and inexplicable. A devastating event in their family caused Drs. Protonotarios and Tsatsopoulou to leave Athens. The city where they both had studied and worked turned against them and became their nemesis. Moreover, no one among their peers within the Athenian academic community seemed to be interested in supporting the studies of the new syndrome. They moved back to Naxos, where they worked in private practice self-supporting their clinical investigations on families with the new syndrome. They also managed to trace inheritance of the affected families 6 generations back, detecting relationships that confirmed the recessive type of inheritance.

Nomenclature and Genetic Studies

The World Congress of Cardiomyopathies held in Warsaw at the end of September 1993 was a key occasion, as it was there that this disorder was named and first presented to an international audience. Names of diseases should be short and easy to pronounce; both doctors were against the idea of giving one of their names to the disorder. They agreed to "Naxos syndrome," as they were confident that the people of Naxos would never misinterpret this nomenclature.

The key point of presentation in Warsaw was the co-segregation of cutaneous abnormalities with ARVC and the implication of a common, potentially genetic mechanism underlying the apparently different manifestations of the skin and the heart. Drs. Protonotarios and Tsatsopoulou were always firm in medically thinking, that "entities should not be multiplied without necessity"; in other words, all symptoms and signs of a patient's illness should be attributed to the same pathogenetic background, unless proven otherwise.[7] Hence, the Naxos syndrome would be an ideal model for linkage analysis and identification of the pathogenic mutation. That was the basis for the fruitful collaboration with Professor McKenna and the London group, which was initiated on the occasion

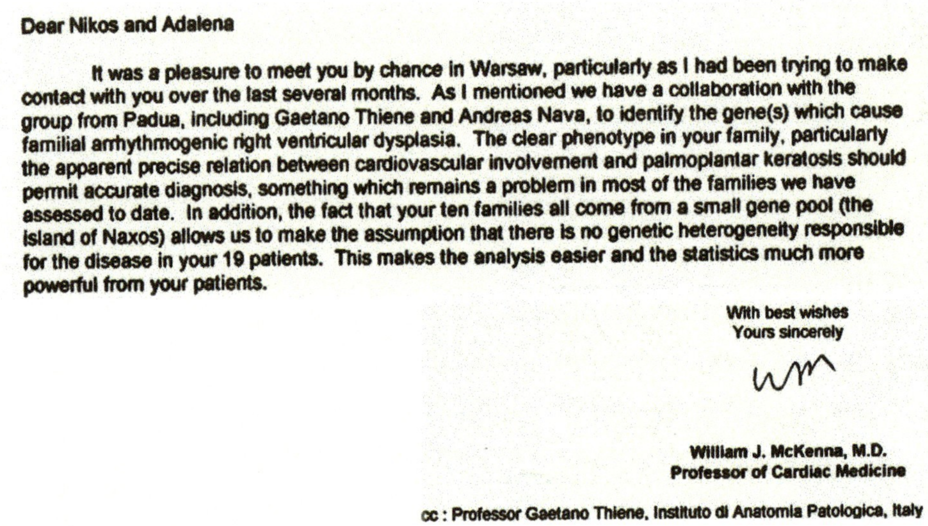

Dear Nikos and Adalena

It was a pleasure to meet you by chance in Warsaw, particularly as I had been trying to make contact with you over the last several months. As I mentioned we have a collaboration with the group from Padua, including Gaetano Thiene and Andreas Nava, to identify the gene(s) which cause familial arrhythmogenic right ventricular dysplasia. The clear phenotype in your family, particularly the apparent precise relation between cardiovascular involvement and palmoplantar keratosis should permit accurate diagnosis, something which remains a problem in most of the families we have assessed to date. In addition, the fact that your ten families all come from a small gene pool (the island of Naxos) allows us to make the assumption that there is no genetic heterogeneity responsible for the disease in your 19 patients. This makes the analysis easier and the statistics much more powerful from your patients.

With best wishes
Yours sincerely

William J. McKenna, M.D.
Professor of Cardiac Medicine

cc : Professor Gaetano Thiene, Instituto di Anatomia Patologica, Italy

FIGURE 1.7 Scanned copy of the letter from Professor McKenna to Drs. Protonotarios and Tsatsopoulou following the initial meetup in Warsaw in 1993 that set the basis for the further collaboration that led to the discovery of the variant causing Naxos disease.

of a Warsaw meeting in 1993 (**Figure 1.7**). The project, apart from sampling the affected persons, included screening of a large number of normal population and family members; people from Naxos and a nearby island, Milos, willingly participated. The gene locus was mapped to 17q21.[8] In the refined region of homozygosity delineating the disease locus, the gene for plakoglobin was located.

A defect in plakoglobin, a constituent protein of desmosomes and adherens junctions, might explain both skin and heart abnormalities since both tissues are subjected to a constant mechanical stress. The fact that the keratoderma of palms and soles was becoming apparent when the affected children started to use their hands and feet supported the candidacy of plakoglobin. Additionally, null plakoglobin mice showed heart and skin abnormalities analogous to Naxos disease.[9] Eventually, a deletion mutation, *Pk2157del2*, was identified to co-segregate with the disease. The mutant protein was also confirmed in cardiac tissue, using a postmortem cardiac biopsy sample, by Western blot analysis using an antiplakoglobin antibody. The findings were published in *The Lancet* in 2000.[10] The Naxos syndrome would ultimately be renamed Naxos disease. It was the first time that an inherited cardiac condition was attributed to a defect in desmosomes. The identification of the *JUP* mutation in Naxos ARVC was a breakthrough in cardiomyopathies, since it paved the way for identification of other desmosomal mutations that underlie the most common nonsyndromic ARVC.

Clinical Projects and Collaborations

In Naxos disease, the first genotype-phenotype study on ARVC was performed and published in 2001.[2] It was quite clear that Naxos ARVC showed 100% penetrance by adolescence, and as a recessive disorder, it was expressing a broad spectrum of the cardiomyopathy phenotype. The disease potential to affect the LV was also revealed; LV involvement detected on echocardiography was documented in 27% of adult patients with Naxos disease.[2] Overcoming conflicts and collaborating is always the key to enable scientists to work together to advance knowledge and discovery in the life sciences. Dr. Protonotarios' priority was sharing data, evaluating patients together with other European experts in ARVC, and designing clinical collaborative studies. So, the clinical expression of *PKP2* and *JUP* mutations was studied in 187 mutation carriers.[11] The two cardiac phenotypes proved to be quite similar, apart from the depolarization changes being more common among patients with Naxos disease, i.e., *JUP* homozygotes. The same study revealed the high sensitivity of precordial repolarization changes and frequent ventricular extrasystoles to clinically detect mutation carriers while it showed the tendency of LV involvement in predisposing to SCD.[11]

Immunohistology demonstrated gap junction remodeling in a collaborative study between Washington University in St. Louis, Missouri, Yannis Protonotarios Medical Centre in Naxos, the University of Athens, the Heart Hospital in London, and Hôpital de la Pitie Salpetriere in Paris. In that study, it was also confirmed for the first time that myocardial gap junction remodeling might exist in ARVC even when no other abnormality on gross pathology or histology can be detected. Furthermore, the abnormal distribution of plakoglobin was the only subcellular defect to underlie the clinical appearance of frequent ventricular ectopics that a child with Naxos cutaneous phenotype presented already at the age of 5 years (**Figure 1.8**).[12]

The long and close clinical follow-up of families with Naxos disease and the existence of cutaneous characteristics from the first year of life permitted early identification of cardiac abnormalities and observation of

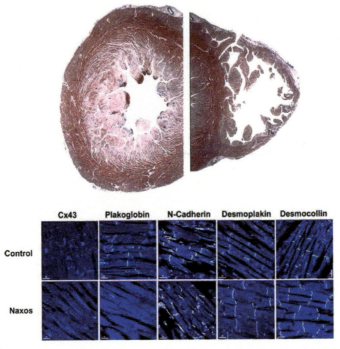

FIGURE 1.8 Histology of the heart showing panoramic transverse sections of the LV and RV, without evidence of fibrofatty replacement (**top**). Representative confocal microscopy images of left ventricle from control and Naxos disease stained with specific antibodies against selected intercellular junction proteins (**bottom**). Cx43 = connexin43. (Figure reproduced from Kaplan et al., *Heart Rhythm.* 2004;1:3–11.[11])

the way that the cardiomyopathy might initiate and progress. Episodes with elevation of cardiac enzymes and documentation of cardiac magnetic resonance late gadolinium enhancement findings suggestive of myocarditis were described as the first clinical presentation or inducing a hot phase in ARVC evolution.[13,14] The reduced arrhythmic potential that advanced ARVC with biventricular dilatation and heart failure might show was demonstrated in a patient with Naxos disease whose heart was also extensively evaluated by the top experts, the team of Professors Gaetano Theine and Cristina Basso in Padua.[15]

In this chapter, only the landmarks in the history of this disorder are described, which is part of the story. The Naxos syndromic association of arrhythmogenic cardiomyopathy with woolly hair and palmoplantar keratoses

is increasingly recognized all over the world. Checking the patient's hands, feet, and hair besides a pure cardiac evaluation brings the patient's care to an improved personalized level. A "hard" feeling while shaking hands with a patient has been established as a warning sign for an underlying arrhythmogenic cardiomyopathy, prompting a more detailed cardiac evaluation of the patient.

References

1. Protonotarios N, Tsatsopoulou A. Naxos disease and Carvajal syndrome: Cardiocutaneous disorders that highlight the pathogenesis and broaden the spectrum of arrhythmogenic right ventricular cardiomyopathy. *Cardiovasc Pathol.* 2004;13(4):185–194. https://doi.org/10.1016/j.carpath.2004.03.609.

2. Protonotarios N, Tsatsopoulou A, Anastasakis A, et al. Genotype-phenotype assessment

in autosomal recessive arrhythmogenic right ventricular cardiomyopathy (Naxos disease) caused by a deletion in plakoglobin. *J Am Coll Cardiol.* 2001;38:1477–1484.

3. Marcus FI, Fontaine GH, Guiraudon G, Frank R, Laurenceau JL, Malergue C, Grosgogeat Y. Right ventricular dysplasia: A report of 24 adult cases. *Circulation.* 1982;65:384–398.

4. Protonotarios N, Tsatsopoulou A, Patsourakos P, Alexopoulos D, Gezerlis P, Simitsis S, Scampardonis G. Cardiac abnormalities in familial palmoplantar keratosis. *Br Heart J.* 1986;56:321–326.

5. Thiene G, Nava A, Corrado D, Rossi L, Pennelli N. Right ventricular cardiomyopathy and sudden death in young people. *N Engl J Med.* 1988;318:129–133.

6. Thiene G, Nava A, Corrado D, Rossi, L, Pennelli N. Right ventricular cardiomyopathy and sudden death in young people [letter]. *N Engl J Med.* 1988;319(3):174–176. doi: 10.1056/NEJM198807213190312.

7. Knowles E. *The Oxford dictionary of phrase and fable.* New York: Oxford University Press, 2005.

8. Coonar AS, Protonotarios N, Tsatsopoulou A, et al. Gene for arrhythmogenic right ventricular cardiomyopathy with diffuse nonepidermolytic palmoplantar keratoderma and woolly hair (Naxos disease) maps to 17q21. *Circulation.* 1998;97:2049–2058.

9. Ruiz P, Brinkmann V, Ledermann B, et al. Targeted mutation of plakoglobin in mice reveals essential functions of desmosomes in the embryonic heart. *J Cell Biol.* 1996;135:215–225.

10. McKoy G, Protonotarios N, Crosby A, et al. Identification of a deletion in plakoglobin in arrhythmogenic right ventricular cardiomyopathy with palmoplantar keratoderma and woolly hair (Naxos disease). *Lancet.* 2000;355:2119–2124.

11. Antoniades L, Tsatsopoulou A, Anastasakis A, et al. Arrhythmogenic right ventricular cardiomyopathy caused by deletions in plakophilin-2 and plakoglobin (Naxos disease) in families from Greece and Cyprus: Genotype-phenotype relations, diagnostic features and prognosis. *Eur Heart J.* 2006;27:2208–2216.

12. Kaplan SR, Gard JJ, Protonotarios N, et al. Remodeling of myocyte gap junctions in arrhythmogenic right ventricular cardiomyopathy due to a deletion in plakoglobin (Naxos disease). *Heart Rhythm.* 2004;1:3–11.

13. Mavrogeni S, Protonotarios N, Tsatsopoulou A, Papachristou P, Sfendouraki E, Papadopoulos G. Naxos disease evolution mimicking acute myocarditis: The role of cardiovascular magnetic resonance imaging. *Int J Cardiol.* 2013;166:e14–e15.

14. Patrianakos AP, Protonotarios N, Nyktari E, Pagonidis K, Tsatsopoulou A, Parthenakis FI, Vardas PE. Arrhythmogenic right ventricular cardiomyopathy/dysplasia and troponin release. Myocarditis or the "hot phase" of the disease? *Int J Cardiol.* 2012;157:e26–e28.

15. Basso C, Tsatsopoulou A, Thiene G, Anastasakis A, Valente M, Protonotarios N. "Petrified" right ventricle in long-standing Naxos arrhythmogenic right ventricular cardiomyopathy. *Circulation.* 2001;104:e132–e133.

2

Metabolic Deregulation in Arrhythmogenic Cardiomyopathy: Novel Pathogenic Insights and Their Clinical Application

Shing Fai Chan, PhD; Liang Chen, MD, PhD; Chuan-yu Wei, PhD; Jiangping Song, MD, PhD; Huei-sheng Vincent Chen, MD, PhD

Introduction

Cardiovascular diseases remain the major cause of death in the world.[1] Recent advances in cellular reprogramming of somatic cells[2-4] from patients with inherited heart diseases into induced pluripotent stem cells (iPSCs) have enabled the generation of cardiomyocytes (CMs) for myocardial repair[5-7] and in vitro modeling of human inherited cardiac diseases.[8-13] However, most published iPSC-based cardiac disease models showed rapid-onset pathologies and exaggerated arrhythmias, frequently occurring spontaneously within 30 days in culture, that deviated greatly from the clinical course of these cardiac diseases.[14-16] Thus, there is a tremendous need to develop more clinically relevant iPSC-CM–based in vitro models for better pathogenic and therapeutic investigations.

Pathologies and Pathogenic Mechanisms of Arrhythmogenic Right Ventricular Cardiomyopathy (ARVC)

ARVC is an inherited cardiomyopathy with most identified mutations in genes that encode cardiac desmosomes, which include plakoglobin (*JUP*), plakophilin-2 (*PKP2*), desmoplakin (*DSP*), desmoglein-2 (*DSG2*), and desmocollin-2 (*DSC2*).[17-21] Pathological hallmarks of ARVC are progressive fibrofatty replacement of CMs with increased CM apoptosis primarily in the right ventricle (RV), leading to heart failure and/or lethal arrhythmias. Clinical criteria to diagnose ARVC are well established,[22] but pathogenic mechanisms of ARVC are difficult to study because obtaining cardiac samples from early stages of human ARVC hearts is rarely possible due to ARVC being commonly diagnosed at advanced disease stages or postmortem. Additionally, primary cardiac tissues are difficult to biopsy safely from symptomatic ARVC patients due to the risk of cardiac perforation. These limiting factors impose significant constraints in developing therapies for human ARVC. Currently, no pathogenesis-guided therapy is available to curtail the progression of ARVC pathologies except standard heart failure therapy, antiarrhythmic medications and ablation to reduce arrhythmia burden, and inserting implantable cardioverter defibrillators (ICDs) to prevent sudden cardiac death (SCD).[22]

How desmosomal mutations could cause CM loss, fibrofatty infiltration, and lethal arrhythmia remains poorly understood. Experimental data from animal and cultured cell line models have led to confusing and conflicting results.[23–28] Early experiments with *DSP* knockdown in murine HL-1 atrial tumor CMs and cardiac-specific *DSP* knockout (KO) mice suggested that *DSP* deficits resulted in aggressive lipogenesis in CMs and nuclear translocation of plakoglobin proteins (JUP). This abnormal JUP nuclear localization was suggested to compete with and decrease the binding of β-catenin to the TCF/LEF transcription factor complexes (gain of function hypothesis), leading to low β-catenin activities and adipogenic transdifferentiation of CMs.[23] However, the majority of human ARVC heart tissues demonstrated significant downregulation of JUP without abnormal nuclear translocation,[24,25] and cardiac-specific KO of *JUP* can reproduce ARVC pathologies in mouse hearts,[26,27] indicating that loss of JUP function, rather than JUP competition with β-catenin, is responsible for eliciting ARVC pathologies.[28] Moreover, *JUP* overexpression can rescue ARVC heart pathologies with JUP deficits, further supporting that loss of JUP function is the pathogenic mechanism for ARVC hearts.[28]

Moreover, using genetic fate mapping techniques in mouse ARVC models, islet-1–positive cardiac progenitor cells of the second heart field have been implicated as the source of adipocytes in ARVC hearts.[29] However, the incorrect use of activation of PPARγ and its target genes as the markers for adipogenesis (adipocyte formation) likely accounted for this misleading interpretation.[23,29] In fact, PPARγ and its target genes are normally activated in several nonadipocyte tissues (e.g., endothelial cells and macrophages)[30] and could be abnormally activated by pathological conditions in hepatocytes (obesity)[31] and CMs (diabetic cardiomyopathy).[32] Therefore, activation of PPARγ and its target genes indicates the active "de novo lipogenesis (DNL)" rather than cell transdifferentiation toward adipocytes. More importantly, the proper lineage marker to identify adipocyte formation (adipogenesis) is perilipin-1 (*PLIN1*) that is only expressed in adipocytes.[33] Also, mesenchymal stromal cells (MSCs) isolated from human ARVC hearts have been shown to be the true source of aggressive adipogenesis in ARVC hearts.[34] In addition, aggressive fibrosis is found in most ARVC hearts and cardiac MSCs are also the main source for aggressive fibrosis in pathological hearts.[35] Thus, the key pathogenic mechanism for exaggerated adipogenic and/or fibrogenic potential of ARVC MSCs remains unresolved.

Establishing iPSCs from Patients with Clinical ARVC and Desmosome Gene Mutations

To further explore the pathogenic mechanisms of human ARVC hearts, we first generated and fully characterized two sets of ARVC *PKP2* mutant iPSC lines from two unrelated ARVC patients.[11] The first ARVC patient has homozygous *PKP2* c.2484C>T mutations[36] with frame-shifted C-terminals that fail to anchor JUP (JK lines), and the other has a heterozygous *PKP2* c.2013delC mutation (delC lines) that causes premature termination codons (leading to a *PKP2* haplo-insufficiency phenotype).[37] We also generated several iPSC lines from normal subjects (CF and WS lines) without any known cardiac disease. First, we find that abnormal nuclear translocation of JUP occurred only in the ARVC iPSC-CMs contacting the rigid plastic culture surface (> 6 gigapascal), indicating that apparent JUP nuclear localization is a culture-induced phenomenon and not a clinically relevant pathological finding.[38] We also find that low β-catenin activity in both *PKP2* mutant ARVC iPSC-CMs at baseline is insufficient for generating ARVC pathologies. Moreover, we did not observe any CM transdifferentiation from human ARVC iPSCs in any culture condition. These results are consistent with the loss-of-function role of JUP in the pathogenesis of ARVC hearts.[28] We now have generated iPSC-CM with mutations in *DSP* or *DSC2* respectively for further pathogenic studies.

Metabolic Maturation-based Pathogenic Induction of ARVC Pathologies

The major metabolic differences between embryonic and adult CMs are (1) embryonic CMs use mainly glycolysis and lactate for energy production, and (2) adult CMs produce most energy via fatty-acid oxidation (FAO) but retain the ability to readily switch to glucose or other substrate utilization when fatty acid is not available or FAO is compromised.[39,40] We first developed a 3-factor (3F) protocol [steroid, insulin, and 3-Isobutyl-1-methylxanthine (IBMX)] to induce PPARα-dependent, adult-like metabolism of cultured iPSC-CMs with significant capacity of FAO but no ARVC pathology. The rationales for designing this 3F metabolic induction protocol had been published in detail.[38] PPARγ is the major transcriptional regulator of fatty-acid metabolism in normal adult CMs.[40] In contrast, PPARγ should be minimally activated in normal CMs. However, the PPARγ pathway has been reported to be abnormally hyperactivated in RV tissue samples of ARVC hearts,[41] and transgene-induced overexpression of PPARγ in mouse CMs could lead to dilated cardiomyopathy.[42] As such, we added to 3F either an endogenous PPARγ agonist 13-hydroxyocta-decadienoic acid (13-HODE, termed 3F+13 HODE) or two strong PPARγ chemical activators (5F protocol = 3F + 5 μM indomethacin and 200 μM rosiglitazone) to activate PPARγ after inducing FAO-dependent metabolism. We found that mutant ARVC iPSC-CMs manifested ARVC pathologies only after induction of adult-like metabolism and abnormal activation of the PPARγ pathway. Coactivation of normal PPARα and abnormal PPARγ pathways resulted in exaggerated lipogenesis, apoptosis, further Na$^+$ channel downregulation,[11,43] and defective intracellular calcium (Ca^{2+}) handling capability in ARVC iPSC-CMs, recapitulating the pathological signatures of ARVC (**Figure 2.1** and see Reference 11), which could be prevented by PPARγ antagonists or overexpression of wildtype (WT) *PKP2* in ARVC iPSC-CMs.[11]

Moreover, based on our functional assays using the Seahorse XF96 Extracellular Flux Analyzer, we observed that the absolute levels of FAO in ARVC iPSC-CMs are always 1.5- to 2-fold higher than those of normal iPSC-CMs after 3F metabolic maturation induction (**Figure 2.2**). This higher FAO flux in ARVC iPSC-CMs might explain why many patients with desmosomal mutations participated and excelled in endurance sports at younger ages prior to the pathological processes that kicked in at adulthood. However, endurance exercises are known to accelerate the pathological phenotypes of ARVC.[44] The elevated cyclic adenosine monophosphate (cAMP) levels

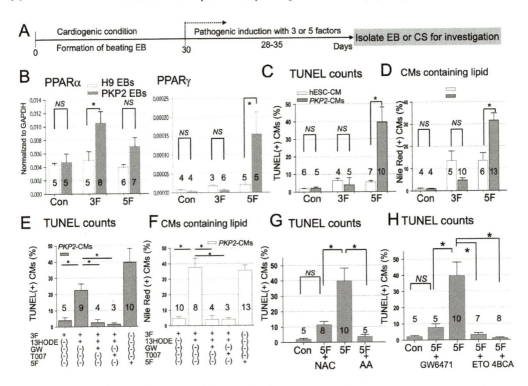

FIGURE 2.1 Metabolic maturation and pathogenic induction of ARVC iPSC-CMs and potential therapeutic strategies. **Panel A:** Protocols for metabolic maturation (3F) and pathogenic (5F) induction. **Panel B:** 3F induced PPARα expression and 5F induced abnormal PPAR-γ activation only in ARVC iPSC-CMs (relative to GAPDH by quantitative RT-PCR). **Panels C and D:** Degrees of CM apoptosis (TUNEL-positive, **Panel C**) and percentage of lipid-laden (Nile-red positive, **Panel D**) CMs after 0F (Con), 3F, or 5F treatment for 4 weeks. **Panels E and F:** Summary of (**Panel E**) degrees of apoptosis and (**Panel F**) lipid-laden CMs in beating embryoid bodies (EBs) is shown here. 13-HODE can replace the indomethacin and rosiglitazone in the 5F protocol to induce ARVC pathologies, which could be prevented by PPAR-γ antagonists, 3 μM GW9662 (GW), or 0.5 μM T0070907 (T007); ROS scavengers, 1 mM N-acetyl-cysteine (NAC), or ascorbic acid (AA; **Panel G**); or scaling down FAO by 2 μM Etomoxir (ETO) or 5 μM 4-bromocrotonic acid (4-BCA; **Panel H**). The number in each column represents the number of biological replicates tested. **Asterisks** indicate $P < 0.05$ and NS, no significant difference by analysis of variance (ANOVA). All data are shown as mean ± SEM. (This figure is adapted from Kim et al., *Nature*. 2013;494:105–110.[11])

from the continuous presence of IBMX in our 3F or 5F protocols likely simulate endurance exercise in real life. We therefore hypothesized that this high FAO flux might also account for the high reactive oxygen species (ROS) production in ARVC iPSC-CMs and is required to drive them toward the apoptotic state after PPARα/PPARγ coactivation. As such, we toned down FAO hyper-flux by adding an EC50 dose of either etomoxir (ETO, to block CPT-1) or 4-bromocrotonic acid (4BCA, to block β-oxidation), which reduced CM apoptosis (Figure 2.1, Panel H). This result strongly supports the use of β-blockers and the recommendation of avoidance of endurance or competitive sports[22] so as to reduce the metabolic flux and the progression of ARVC phenotypes.

Plasma β-OHB Levels Predict Adverse Outcomes and Pathological Disease Progression in ARVC

The onset of clinical symptoms/signs of ARVC is usually unpredictable. The clinically concealed phase of ARVC, even in individuals

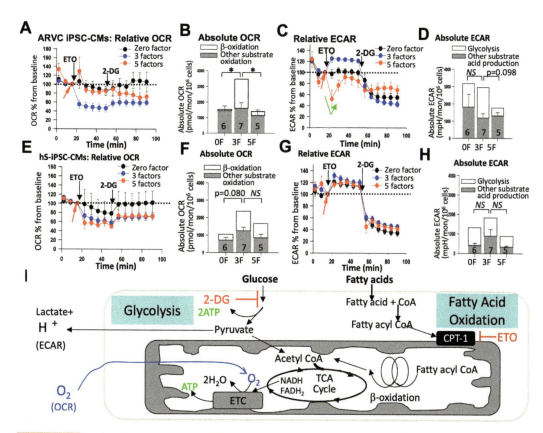

FIGURE 2.2 Functional assays of glucose utilization versus FAO in *PKP2* mutant iPSC-CMs after various treatments. Using a Seahorse XF96 Extracellular Flux Analyzer, we determined the degree of FAO by measuring the etomoxir (100 µM ETO, a specific CPT-1 inhibitor) blocked components of OCR, and glycolysis by measuring 2-deoxyglucose (50 mM 2-DG) blocked components of ECAR (see Reference 11 for detailed methods). Absolute values of OCR and ECAR are expressed as pmol/min/10^6 cells and mpH/min/10^6 cells, respectively. **Panel A:** Real-time measurement of OCR showed that ETO blocked 14.4 ± 10.2 (0F), 53.9 ± 8.2 (3F), and 15.3 ± 8.5% (5F) of baseline OCR (**red arrow**) for ARVC iPSC-CMs. **Panel B:** ETO-blocked absolute OCR (**white boxes**) for ARVC iPSC-CMs are 85.2 ± 196.6 (0F), 1865.3 ± 383.5 (3F), and 254.5 ± 115.4 (5F). **Panel C:** ECAR measurement after ETO inhibition of β-oxidation showed a rapid ~21% compensatory increase of glycolysis only in the 3F condition (a switch in energy substrates); yet, after 5F, ETO transiently decreased ECAR by ~45% (**green arrow**) followed by ~28% compensatory increase in ECAR (glycolysis). **Panel D:** 2DG-blocked absolute ECAR (glycolysis) for ARVC iPSC-CMs after 0F, 3F or 5F are 1353.0 ± 313.6, 1766.0 ± 579.7, and 457.2 ± 211.0, respectively. Comparable patterns in absolute and relative OCR or ECAR in normal hS-iPSC-CMs (WS#4) are shown (**Panel E–H**). For normal iPSC-CMs, ETO-blocked FAO after 0F, 3F, or 5F are (**Panel E**) (relative) 21.8 ± 24.8%, 42.6 ± 6.6%, and 50.5 ± 4.06%; or (**Panel F**) (absolute) 329.4 ± 235.8, 1114.5 ± 316.6, and 807.8 ± 196.4, respectively. 2DG-blocked glycolysis after 0F, 3F, or 5F are (**Panel G**) (relative) 65.5 ± 5.3%, 54.9 ± 3.8%, and 58.8 ± 4.8%; or (**Panel H**) (absolute) 915.3 ± 270.6, 929.4 ± 314.3, and 556.8 ± 217.9, respectively. **Panel I:** A simple diagram to illustrate substrate utilization pathways in CMs. These results (**Panels A–H**) support that both normal and ARVC iPSC-CMs 1) display embryonic metabolism at baseline, and 2) show significantly increases FAO after 3F with ability to switch between FAO and glucose utilization (an adult-like metabolic pattern). ARVC iPSC-CMs after 5F behave like failing CMs with pathological burnt-out metabolism. Single asterisk indicates *p* < 0.05 and *NS*, no significant difference by ANOVA. *P* values are shown when unpaired *t*-test was performed. (This figure is adapted from Kim et al., *Nature.* 2013;494:105–110.[11])

with known mutations, could last 20 to 40 years, and some patients' relatives could be asymptomatic carriers. Unfortunately, SCD could be the first symptom of patients with ARVC. The progression of ARVC is not predictable and could have flares of "hot" phases with malignant ventricular arrhythmias (VAs) and heart failure.[17–22] Thus, establishing a biomarker for early diagnosis and better risk stratification[45] of ARVC patients and their relatives[46] is quintessential for preventing SCD in patients with ARVC. Current diagnosis and risk stratification have focused largely on clinically detectable changes in arrhythmia burden and abnormalities of cardiac structure and function.[45–47] Serum markers, such as C-reactive protein and N-terminal pro-B type natriuretic peptide, have been reported to associate with ARVC. However, these serum markers are routinely used for general evaluation of cardiac dysfunction and are not specific for ARVC or predictive of malignant arrhythmias in patients with ARVC.[48,49]

Since ARVC iPSC-CMs displayed higher levels of FAO than normal iPSC-CMs (Figure 2.2) at mature and prediseased states, we hypothesized that metabolic markers of increased FAO in early-stage ARVC hearts may provide clues for early diagnosis of ARVC and that markers of FAO-related metabolic abnormalities may be used as predictors for adverse disease progression of ARVC hearts. Because ketone production and utilization are closely associated with high FAO and extra-hepatic lipogenesis,[50] we measured β-hydroxybutyrate (β-OHB, a major form of ketones in human plasma) concentrations from culture media and CM lysates of ARVC iPSC-CMs after 3F metabolic maturation induction and 5F pathological induction (**Figure 2.3**, Panels A and B).[51] The assays demonstrated a significant increase in β-OHB production from pathological ARVC CMs and release into culture medium at early stages (1 week, $P < 0.05$) and returned to baseline levels at an intermediate pathological stage when CMs started showing apoptosis and impaired FAO at 2.5 weeks (Figure 2.3, Panels C and D). Seahorse metabolic assays showed that ARVC iPSC-CMs at 2 weeks after pathological induction already displayed decreased overall oxidative phosphorylation, and at 4 weeks of pathological induction they had very low long-chain fatty acid (LCFA) oxidation with increased utilization of other metabolic substrates for oxidative phosphorylation (Figure 2.3, Panels C and D). The ketogenesis process after 2 weeks of 5F treatment was significantly diminished owing to the decreased FAO of LCFA shown by Seahorse metabolic assays.

The results in Figure 2.3 support that ARVC CMs likely are ketogenic from high FAO at early prepathological stages in vitro. Thus, we measured the plasma β-OHB levels of the first- and second-degree relatives of 65 ARVC probands. We classified ARVC probands' relatives who had syncope or were positive for at least one of the ARVC Task Force Criteria (TFC) in echocardiography or electrocardiography (ECG) studies as suspected ARVC relatives or early-phase patients (n = 25). We found that plasma β-OHB levels of suspected ARVC relatives are higher than those of unaffected relatives (n = 69; fold change = 1.52, $P < 0.001$; **Figure 2.4**, Panel A), whereas unaffected relatives had the same plasma β-OHB levels as healthy volunteers. A receiver-operating characteristic (ROC) curve analysis showed that plasma β-OHB could distinguish suspected ARVC relatives from unaffected relatives with a sensitivity of 56.00% and a specificity of 93.94% using a cutoff value of 30.76 μM (AUC = 0.783, $P < 0.001$). Thus, plasma β-OHB levels could be used as an early diagnostic marker of adverse disease progression in relatively asymptomatic ARVC relatives with excellent specificity.

We next investigated whether the presence of heart failure or history of arrhythmia correlated with plasma β-OHB levels in

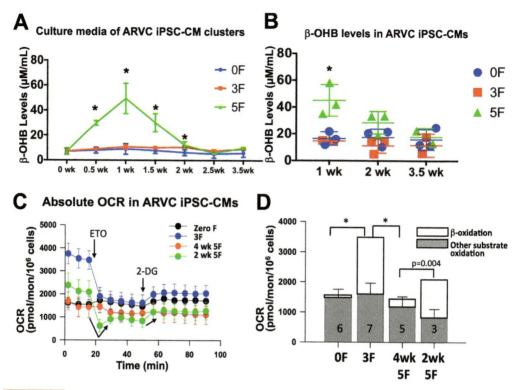

FIGURE 2.3 Increased ketone (β-OHB) production (ketogenesis) with high FAO at early stages, and later decreased FAO with no more ketone production at intermediate to advanced stages after pathogenic induction by 5F in ARVC CMs, is presented. ARVC iPSC-CMs treated with 5F showed increased β-OHB levels in both culture media (**Panel A**) and CMs (**Panel B**) at 1–2 weeks, preceding the irreversible ARVC pathologies at 2.5–4 weeks. **Panel C:** Using real-time Seahorse XF96 metabolic flux measurement, 5F treated ARVC iPSC-CMs at 2 weeks show decreased overall oxidative phosphorylation, and the small compensatory increases of OCR after ETO and 2-DG treatment indicate the compensatory increases in utilization of other metabolic substrates for oxidative phosphorylation. **Panel D:** 5F treated ARVC iPSC-CMs at 4 weeks are at a metabolic burnt-out state and rely on other metabolic substrates for oxidative phosphorylation. (This figure is adapted from Kim et al., *Nature.* 2013;494:105–110[11] and Song et al., *Sci Transl Med.* 2020;12:eaay8329.[51])

patients with ARVC. In 65 ARVC probands, plasma β-OHB levels of patients with biventricular heart failure (n = 12), with isolated RV failure (n = 30), or with only VAs (n = 23) are higher than those of 56 healthy volunteers (Figure 2.4, Panel B). Thirty-four of 65 ARVC patients had major adverse cardiovascular events (MACE), defined as those who had syncope, sustained VA, appropriate ICD shocks, or heart transplant (HTx), and their plasma β-OHB levels are higher than those of ARVC patients without MACE (Figure 2.4, Panel C). Of note, no cardiac dysfunction-dependent elevation of β-OHB was observed (see Reference 51 for detailed data). These results support that plasma β-OHB levels in patients with ARVC are elevated early and before RV or left ventricular (LV) failure and that elevation of plasma β-OHB levels is not a compensatory response of heart failure but rather a specific metabolic signature in patients with ARVC. Thus, plasma β-OHB levels in patients with ARVC and their relatives might be an early biomarker of adverse pathological progression in ARVC. To explore whether plasma β-OHB levels could serve as an indicator of disease progression over the entire ARVC disease spectrum, we categorized ARVC pathological progression and corresponding plasma β-OHB levels into

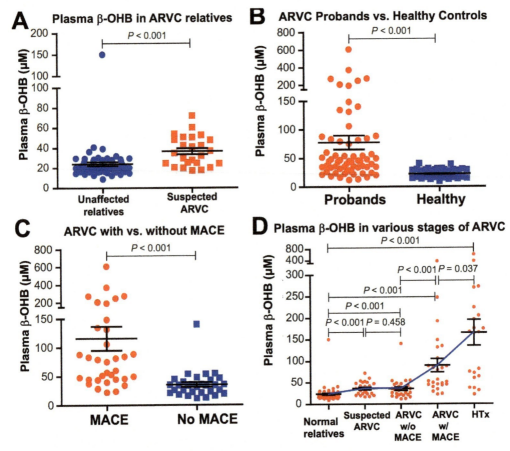

FIGURE 2.4 Plasma β-OHB levels rise with the adverse progression of the ARVC pathological processes. **Panel A:** Plasma β-OHB levels are higher in ARVC relatives with some ARVC diagnostic criteria than those of completely unaffected relatives. **Panel B:** In general, ARVC probands have higher plasma β-OHB levels than healthy controls. **Panel C:** In ARVC probands, patients with major adverse cardiac events (MACE) have higher plasma β-OHB levels than probands without MACE. **Panel D:** Progressive increases in plasma β-OHB levels stratified by five progressively worsening stages of ARVC according to clinical presentation and MACE events [unaffected relatives, suspected ARVC, ARVC without MACE, ARVC with MACE, and ARVC patients requiring HTx].

5 progressively worsening stages according to clinical presentation and MACE events, from completely unaffected relatives (24.04 ± 2.00 μM, n = 69), suspected ARVC (36.47 ± 2.98 μM, n = 25), early ARVC [ARVC patients without MACE (35.48 ± 4.11 μM, n = 31)], advanced ARVC [ARVC probands with MACE but no need for HTx, 89.82 ± .43 μM, n = 26], to end-stage ARVC who received HTx during follow-up (165.60 ± 30.23 μM, n = 21). Plasma β-OHB levels increased progressively with the severity of the disease (Figure 2.4, Panel D), supporting that progressively rising plasma β-OHB levels in patients with ARVC and their relatives indicate underlying adverse disease progression. Thus, we demonstrate that cardiac ketogenesis occurs in early ARVC CMs. Plasma β-OHB levels could be used as a potential biomarker to predict not only MACE in ARVC probands but also disease progression in ARVC patients and their family members, particularly useful for individuals at the concealed phase.

Distinct Metabolic Phenotypes of Immature, Mature, and Pathological ARVC CMs

Using the Seahorse XF96 Extracellular Flux Analyzer,[52] functional assays of FAO and glycolysis in live cells revealed that normal and ARVC iPSC-CMs had dominant glycolytic energetics (an embryonic pattern) at baseline (Figure 2.2, Panels A–H). After activation of PPARα by 3F, mutant and normal iPSC-CMs displayed slightly higher levels of glycolysis but significant activation of FAO (an adult-like pattern) when compared to the un-induced, baseline conditions [zero factor (0F)]. Compared to 3F induction, mutant *PKP2* iPSC-CMs treated with 5F for 4 weeks, demonstrated overall depressed energy metabolism with more FAO reduction (from using LCFA) than the reduction in glycolysis, resulting in a fuel shift from using both fatty acids and glucose to primarily glucose utilization (including glycolysis and pyruvate oxidation) and other substrate oxidation, much like the so-called metabolic burnt-out state observed in failing hearts (**Figure 2.5**).[53] More importantly, our metabolomic analysis[51] indicates that the end-stage ARVC human hearts depict impaired LCFA utilization and elevated utilization of medium-chain fatty acid (MCFA) without increased ketone utilization, an unique metabolic pattern that differs from metabolic burnt-out phenotypes in other types of dilated cardiomyopathy.[51]

Conclusions and Future Perspective

Using patient-specific mutant *PKP2* iPSC-CMs grown in a 3D beating EB format and induced by various maturation/pathogenic conditions, we accelerate the pathogenesis of an adult-onset cardiac disease. We demonstrate the importance of PPARα-dependent/adult-like metabolism, PPARγ coactivation, ROS production, and high flux of fatty acid oxidation in the pathogenesis of ARVC.[11] This efficient in vitro iPSC-CM–based model recapitulates the pathognomonic features of ARVC hearts and enables pathogenic investigation and therapeutic screens. Future research to elucidate how mutant *PKP2* leads to abnormal PPARγ activation in ARVC CMs would further deepen our understanding of this unfortunate disease and pave the way for developing novel therapeutics.

Furthermore, we observed increased ketogenesis in early ARVC CMs that could be used to diagnose adverse pathological progression of ARVC relatives in the fairly asymptomatic stages. More importantly, we find that plasma β-OHB levels in ARVC probands correlate well with the adverse disease progressions. Finally, metabolic and metabolomic assays show that both end-stage explanted ARVC hearts and pathological ARVC iPSC-CMs are in a metabolic burnt-out state with MCFAs as the main energy fuel. Thus, using in vitro iPSC-CM model and *in vivo* explanted ARVC diseased hearts, we reveal that metabolic derangement is the main pathogenic mechanism of ARVC hearts. Future prospective clinical trials using plasma β-OHB (ketones) levels to diagnose adverse disease progression in asymptomatic ARVC relatives, and ARVC probands are needed to support our pathogenic findings and to confirm the usefulness of plasma β-OHB (ketones) levels as the diagnostic marker for adverse disease progression in ARVC. Also, we must devote effort and time into studying the mechanisms of CM maturation so as to build better and more clinically relevant in-vitro models before an applicable therapeutic screen can be pursued.

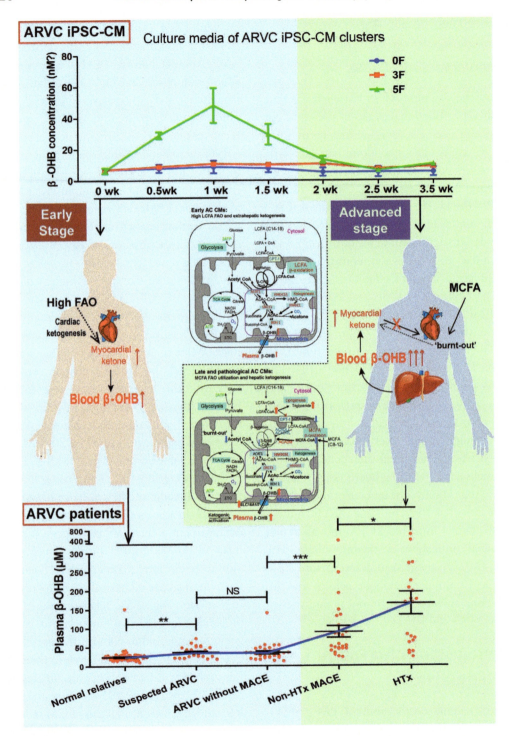

FIGURE 2.5 Summary scheme for ketone body metabolism and metabolic deregulations in early and advanced stages of ARVC. In early or relatively asymptomatic stages of ARVC, ARVC CMs are ketogenic and producing β-OHB that could be used to diagnose adverse disease progression in ARVC relatives. In the intermediate and late stages of ARVC, ARVC CMs show decreased FAO and no ketone production, leading to progressive accumulation of plasma ketones (produced by the liver) that could be used to predict MACE in ARVC probands.

Acknowledgments

We thank the patients for their participation, microarray core facilities at Sanford-Burnham-Prebys Medical Discovery Institute (SBP) for their support, the Johns Hopkins ARVC registry for their valuable support, and George W. Rogers from Seahorse Bioscience for assistance in metabolic assays. Huei-sheng Vincent Chen was supported by grants from the National Institutes of Health and Krannert Institute of Cardiology Start-up Funds.

The authors report no conflicts of interest in relation to this article.

References

1. Go AS, Mozaffarian D, Roger VL, et al. Heart disease and stroke statistics–2014 update: A report from the American Heart Association. *Circulation.* 2014;129:e28–e292.

2. Takahashi K, Tanabe K, Ohnuki M, et al. Induction of pluripotent stem cells from adult human fibroblasts by defined factors. *Cell.* 2007;131:861–872.

3. Yu J, Vodyanik MA, Smuga-Otto K, et al. Induced pluripotent stem cell lines derived from human somatic cells. *Science.* 2007;318:1917–1920.

4. Park IH, Arora N, Huo H, et al. Disease-specific induced pluripotent stem cells. *Cell.* 2008;134:877–886.

5. Okano H, Nakamura M, Yoshida K, et al. Steps toward safe cell therapy using induced pluripotent stem cells. *Circ Res.* 2013;112:523–533.

6. Shiba Y, Fernandes S, Zhu WZ, et al. Human ES-cell-derived cardiomyocytes electrically couple and suppress arrhythmias in injured hearts. *Nature.* 2012;489:322–325.

7. Chen HS, Kim C, Mercola M. Electrophysiological challenges of cell-based myocardial repair. *Circulation.* 2009;120:2496–2508.

8. Carvajal-Vergara X, Sevilla A, D'Souza SL, et al. Patient-specific induced pluripotent stem-cell-derived models of LEOPARD syndrome. *Nature.* 2010;465:808–812.

9. Itzhaki I, Maizels L, Huber I, et al. Modelling the long QT syndrome with induced pluripotent stem cells. *Nature.* 2011;471:225–229.

10. Moretti A, Laugwitz KL, Dorn T, Sinnecker D, Mummery C. Pluripotent stem cell models of human heart disease. *Cold Spring Harbor Persp Med.* 2013;3(11).

11. Kim C, Wong J, Wen J, et al. Studying arrhythmogenic right ventricular dysplasia with patient-specific iPSCs. *Nature.* 2013;494:105–110.

12. Mercola M, Colas A, Willems E. Induced pluripotent stem cells in cardiovascular drug discovery. *Circ Res.* 2013;112:534–548.

13. Shinnawi R, Gepstein L. iPSC cell modeling of inherited cardiac arrhythmias. *Curr Treat Options Cardiovasc Med.* 2014;16:331.

14. Yang X, Pabon L, Murry CE. Engineering adolescence: Maturation of human pluripotent stem cell-derived cardiomyocytes. *Circ Res.* 2014;114:511–523.

15. Veerman CC, Kosmidis G, Mummery CL, Casini S, Verkerk AO, Bellin M. Immaturity of human stem-cell-derived cardiomyocytes in culture: Fatal flaw or soluble problem? *Stem Cells Dev.* 2015;24:1035–1052.

16. Santostefano KE, Hamazaki T, Biel NM, Jin S, Umezawa A, Terada N. A practical guide to induced pluripotent stem cell research using patient samples. *Lab Invest.* 2015;95:4–13.

17. Marcus FI, Fontaine GH, Guiraudon G, et al. Right ventricular dysplasia: A report of 24 adult cases. *Circulation.* 1982;65:384–398.

18. Calkins H. Arrhythmogenic right ventricular dysplasia/cardiomyopathy—three decades of progress. *Circ J.* 2015;79:901–913.

19. den Haan AD, Tan BY, Zikusoka MN, et al. Comprehensive desmosome mutation analysis in North Americans with arrhythmogenic right ventricular dysplasia/cardiomyopathy. *Circ Cardiovasc Genet.* 2009;2:428–435.

20. Awad MM, Calkins H, Judge DP. Mechanisms of disease: Molecular genetics of arrhythmogenic right ventricular dysplasia/cardiomyopathy. *Nat Clin Pract Cardiovasc Med.* 2008;5:258–267.

Note: A more comprehensive description is reported in Dr. Fontaine's book (in French). It is cited as the last bibliographic reference of this chapter.

21. Basso C, Bauce B, Corrado D, Thiene G. Pathophysiology of arrhythmogenic cardiomyopathy. *Nat Rev Cardiol.* 2012;9:223–233.

22. Marcus FI, McKenna WJ, Sherrill D, et al. Diagnosis of arrhythmogenic right ventricular cardiomyopathy/dysplasia: Proposed modification of the Task Force Criteria. *Eur Heart J.* 2010;31:806–814.

23. Garcia-Gras, E, Lombardi R, Giocondo MJ, et al. Suppression of canonical Wnt/beta-catenin signaling by nuclear plakoglobin recapitulates phenotype of arrhythmogenic right ventricular cardiomyopathy. *J Clin Invest.* 2006;116:2012–2021.

24. Asimaki A, Tandri H, Huang H, et al. A new diagnostic test for arrhythmogenic right ventricular cardiomyopathy. *N Engl J Med.* 2009;360:1075–1084.

25. Basso C, Pilichou K, Thiene G. Is it time for plakoglobin immune-histochemical diagnostic test for arrhythmogenic cardiomyopathy in the routine pathology practice? *Cardiovasc Pathol.* 2013;22:312–313.

26. Li D, Liu Y, Maruyama M, et al. Restrictive loss of plakoglobin in cardiomyocytes leads to arrhythmogenic cardiomyopathy. *Hum Mol Genet.* 2011;20:4582–4596.

27. Swope D, Cheng L, Gao E, Li J, Radice GL. Loss of cadherin-binding proteins β-catenin and plakoglobin in the heart leads to gap junction remodeling and arrhythmogenesis. *Mol Cell Biol.* 2012;32:1056–1067.

28. Zhang Z, Stroud MJ, Zhang J, et al. Normalization of Naxos plakoglobin levels restores cardiac function in mice. *J Clin Invest.* 2015;125:1708–1712.

29. Lombardi R, Dong J, Rodriguez G, et al. Genetic fate mapping identifies second heart field progenitor cells as a source of adipocytes in arrhythmogenic right ventricular cardiomyopathy. *Circ Res.* 2009;104:1076–1084.

30. Wilson TM, Lambert MH, Kliewer SA. Peroxisome proliferator-activated receptor gamma and metabolic disease. *Annu Rev Biochem.* 2001;70:341–367.

31. Pettinelli P, Videla LA. Up-regulation of PPAR-gamma mRNA expression in the liver of obese patients: An additional reinforcing lipogenic mechanism to SREBP-1c induction. *J Clin Endocrinol Metab.* 2011;96:1424–1430.

32. Marfella R, Portoghese M, Ferraraccio F, et al. Thiazolidinediones may contribute to the intramyocardial lipid accumulation in diabetic myocardium: Effects on cardiac function. *Heart.* 2009;95:1020–1022.

33. Brasaemle DL. Thematic review series: Adipocyte biology. The perilipin family of structural lipid droplet proteins: Stabilization of lipid droplets and control of lipolysis. *J Lipid Res.* 2007;48:2547–2559.

34. Sommariva E, Brambilla S, Carbucicchio C, et al. Cardiac mesenchymal stromal cells are a source of adipocytes in arrhythmogenic cardiomyopathy. *Eur Heart J.* 2016;37:1835–1846.

35. El Agha E, Kramann R, Schneider RK, et al. Mesenchymal stem cells in fibrotic disease. *Cell Stem Cell.* 2017;21:166–177.

36. Awad MM, Dalal D, Tichnell C, et al. Recessive arrhythmogenic right ventricular dysplasia due to novel cryptic splice mutation in PKP2. *Hum Mutat.* 2006;27:1157.

37. Dalal D, Molin LH, Piccini J, et al. Clinical features of arrhythmogenic right ventricular dysplasia/cardiomyopathy associated with mutations in plakophilin-2. *Circulation.* 2006;113:1641–1649.

38. Shah K, Wei CY, Kim C, et al. Modelling arrhythmogenic right ventricular dysplasia/cardiomyopathy with patient-specific iPSCs. In: Fukuda K, ed., *Human iPS Cells in Disease Modelling.* Springer, 2016;Chapter 3:27–43.

39. Onay-Besikci A. Regulation of cardiac energy metabolism in newborn. *Mol Cell Biochem.* 2006;287:1–11.

40. Lopaschuk GD, Ussher JR, Folmes CD, Jaswal JS, Stanley WC. Myocardial fatty acid metabolism in health and disease. *Physiol Rev.* 2010;90:207–258.

41. Djouadi F, Lecarpentier Y, Hebert JL, Charron P, Bastin J, Coirault C. A potential link between peroxisome proliferator-activated receptor signalling and the pathogenesis of arrhythmogenic right ventricular cardiomyopathy. *Cardiovasc Res.* 2009;84:83–90.

42. Son NH, Park TS, Yamashita H, et al. Cardiomyocyte expression of PPARgamma leads to cardiac dysfunction in mice. *J Clin Invest.* 2007;117:2791–2801.

43. Cerrone M, Lin X, Zhang M, et al. Missense mutations in plakophilin-2 cause sodium current deficit and associate with a Brugada syndrome phenotype. *Circulation.* 2014;129:1092–1103.

44. Sawant AC, Bhonsale A, te Riele AS, et al. Exercise has a disproportionate role in the pathogenesis of arrhythmogenic right ventricular dysplasia/cardiomyopathy in patients without desmosomal mutations. *J Am Heart Assoc.* 2014;3:e001471.

45. Calkins H, Corrado D, Marcus F. Risk stratification in arrhythmogenic right ventricular cardiomyopathy. *Circulation.* 2017;136:2068–2082.

46. te Riele AS, James CA, Groeneweg JA, et al. Approach to family screening in arrhythmogenic right ventricular dysplasia/cardiomyopathy. *Eur. Heart J.* 2016;37:755–763.

47. Cadrin-Tourigny J, Bosman LP, Nozza A, et al. A new prediction model for ventricular arrhythmias in arrhythmogenic right ventricular cardiomyopathy. *Eur Heart J.* 2019;40:1850–1858.

48. Scharhag J, Urhausen A, Schneider G, et al. Reproducibility and clinical significance of exercise-induced increases in cardiac troponins and N-terminal pro brain natriuretic peptide in endurance athletes. *Eur J Cardiovasc Prev Rehabil.* 2006;13:388–397.

49. Bonny A, Lellouche N, Ditah I, et al. C-reactive protein in arrhythmogenic right ventricular dysplasia/cardiomyopathy and relationship with ventricular tachycardia. *Cardiol Res Pract.* 2010;2010:919783.

50. Cotter DG, Schugar RC, Crawford PA. Ketone body metabolism and cardiovascular disease. *Am J Physiol Heart Circ Physiol.* 2013;304:H1060–H1076.

51. Song JP, Chen L, Chen X, et al. Elevated plasma-hydroxybutyrate predicts adverse outcomes and disease progression in patients with arrhythmogenic cardiomyopathy. *Sci Transl Med.* 2020;12:eaay8329.

52. Ferrick DA, Neilson A, Beeson C. Advances in measuring cellular bioenergetics using extracellular flux. *Drug Discov Today.* 2008;13:268–274.

53. Neubauer S. The failing heart—an engine out of fuel. *N Engl J Med.* 2007;356:1140–1151.

3

Pleiotropic Functions of Plakophilin-2 and Arrhythmia Mechanisms

Marina Cerrone, MD; Chantal J. M. van Opbergen, PhD; Mario Delmar, MD, PhD

Introduction

Arrhythmogenic cardiomyopathy (ACM, also referred to as arrhythmogenic right ventricular cardiomyopathy, or ARVC) is an inheritable condition characterized by a fibrofatty infiltration of the heart muscle, as well as increased risk of ventricular arrhythmias (VAs) and sudden cardiac death (SCD).[1–3] The disease phenotype progresses over time, with lethal arrhythmias often observed in the early stages before the onset of the cardiomyopathy. The structural disease most commonly (though not always) starts in the right ventricular (RV) free wall, later involving the left ventricle (LV) and ultimately resulting in biventricular heart failure.[1,3] Its prevalence is estimated at around 1:2000–1:5000 and it is considered one of the predominant causes of unexpected SCD in athletes.[4,5] Mutations in genes coding for cardiac desmosomal proteins account for most familial cases with known genetic sub-strate, with the gene *PKP2*, coding for pla-kophilin-2 (PKP2), being the most commonly involved.[6,7] Desmosomal proteins have a clear role in cell–cell adhesion; hence it has been postulated that defective desmosomes could promote fibrosis by weakening intercellular adhesion strength between cardiomyocytes (CMs).[8,9] However, this hypothesis could not easily justify some other aspects of ACM, such as the known adipose infiltration of the cardiac tissue or the arrhythmogenic phenotype observed in the precardiomyopathic stages. Recent data from our group and others[10–12] have shown that defective or deficient PKP2 in the context of ACM can alter multiple molecular pathways and lead to transcriptional modifications, thus encompassing a wider spectrum of functions in addition to the one related to cell–cell adhesion. In this chapter we will review the pleiotropic aspects of PKP2 loss at the molecular level and their relation to the ACM phenotype.

25

A Novel Mouse Model of PKP2 Haploinsufficiency

Engineered mouse models are a valuable tool to unravel molecular mechanisms of inherited arrhythmogenic conditions, even given the obvious limitations of an animal system that does not recapitulate all aspects of the human disease. Mice with global *PKP2* knockout die during gestation.[13] The germline heterozygous *PKP2* knockout mouse is viable and reaches adulthood; yet it only presents arrhythmias and ultrastructural changes, without developing a real cardiomyopathy.[14,15] We then generated a cardiac-specific, tamoxifen-activated *PKP2* knockout murine line (PKP2-cKO).[10] This mouse model starts developing an RV dilation about 14 days postinjection (DPI) of tamoxifen (mice are injected when they are 3–4 months of age), then develops an RV cardiomyopathy and ultimately progresses into LV dilation and end-stage heart failure between 28 and 42 DPI (**Figure 3.1**). Histological signs of fibrosis are apparent after 21 DPI in the RV, when the LV is still mostly spared.

Interestingly, the PKP2-cKO mouse has also high propensity for adrenergic-induced VAs. Spontaneous and isoproterenol-induced ventricular arrhythmias and lethal ventricular fibrillation are observed around 16 to 21 DPI in anesthetized mice, thus before the onset of overt structural cardiomyopathy.

Transcriptional Changes Linked to PKP2 Deficiency Alter Cardiac Calcium Cycling

PKP2 is a protein of the connexome, residing at the intercalated disc and scaffolding an intracellular signaling hub linked to multiple molecular pathways.[16–18] Dysfunction of this hub leads to an expanding chain of events that disrupts the transcriptional program. Transcriptome changes associated with defective PKP2 have been evaluated in the context of fibro-adipogenic genes.[12,19] Using the PKP2-cKO mouse model, we investigated transcriptomic changes occurring in the adult heart after loss of PKP2 expression in the cardiac tissue that may impact arrhythmogenesis. We

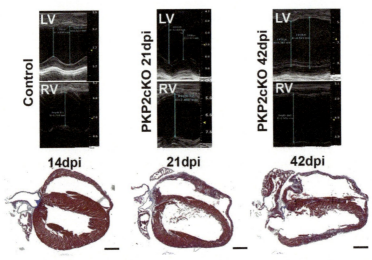

FIGURE 3.1   Timeline progression of the cardiac phenotype in the PKO2-cKO mouse is shown. **Upper panels:** M-mode echocardiogram images are presented of LV and RV in control (**left**), PKP2-cKO hearts at 21 DPI (**middle**), and 42 DPI (**right**). **Bottom panels:** Histology sections with Masson-trichrome staining of LV and RV at 14 DPI (**left**), 221 DPI (**middle**), and 42 DPI (**right**) show progression from a structurally intact heart, RV-only dilation and fibrosis, and biventricular dilation and fibrosis, respectively. (Reproduced with permission from Cerrone et al., *Nat Commun.* 2017;8:106.[10])

performed RNA-seq from PKP2-cKO mouse hearts and their littermate controls at 21 DPI, choosing hearts with absence of fibrosis. Significant differential expression was observed with 510 transcripts being downregulated and 705 being upregulated.[10] When we focused on the KEGG functional network analysis of the downregulated pathways, it emerged that one of the most relevant pathways was calcium signaling. Of note, isoproterenol- and/or adrenergic-induced arrhythmias resulting from dysregulation of intracellular calcium (Ca^{2+}_i) and triggered activity are seen in other conditions known to have altered Ca^{2+} homeostasis, such as catecholaminergic polymorphic ventricular tachycardia (CPVT).[20,21]

Transcriptional and protein abundance changes resulted in an increase in the amplitude and a prolonged duration of Ca^{2+} transients, leading to occurrence of early and delayed after-transients, evidence of sarcoplasmic reticulum load, and increased amplitude and frequency of spontaneous Ca^{2+} release events. Additionally, optical mapping experiments confirmed prolongation of the Ca^{2+} transients' duration in the isolated Langendorff-perfused mouse heart. Altogether, these data provided a molecular substrate for the arrhythmias detected *in vivo* in the PKP2-cKO mouse in the early disease stage. Based on the evidence that increased sarcoplasmic reticulum load and triggered activity could offer a substrate for lethal arrhythmias in the precardiomyopathic stages, we investigated if flecainide could be an effective therapeutic option. Previous evidence had shown that flecainide exerts a direct RyR2 channel-blocking effect, in addition to the known sodium channel blockade.[22] Indeed, it is a recognized, effective therapy in the setting of CPVT, a disease caused by genetically mediated RyR2 channels leakage.[20,23,24] In addition, few reports had identified *PKP2* mutations in cases of autopsy-negative sudden unexplained death in the young and in patients with initial clinical diagnosis of CPVT and absence of identifiable structural cardiomyopathy.[25] Flecainide treatment completely abolished the occurrence of isoproterenol-induced arrhythmias in the PKP2-cKO mouse, further supporting the notion that arrhythmias in the early stages of the disease could be the result of dysregulation of Ca^{2+}_i cycling via increased RyR2-dependent Ca^{2+} release.

Anecdotal successful use of flecainide in patients with ACM was also recently reported.[26] Although there are obvious differences between a mouse model of PKP2 haploinsufficiency and the human condition, these data provided a solid background for the first ongoing prospective randomized clinical trial evaluating the effect of flecainide in the setting of ACM in the United States (NCT03685149).

Right Versus Left Ventricular Asymmetry in ACM and Arrhythmias

Even if it is recognized that ACM is a condition that can involve both ventricular chambers, it is also known that the disease starts manifesting as an RV-predominant cardiomyopathy in the majority of cases with a *PKP2* mutation.

Furthermore, lethal VAs can occur in hearts with *PKP2* mutations before the RV structural involvement becomes detectable.[25] We took advantage of the PKP2-cKO model to identify the earliest molecular signals that can be detected prior to the overt phenotype. Analysis of hearts 16 days post-tamoxifen injection (16 DPI) revealed the occurrence of adrenergic-induced arrhythmias, with a few animals experiencing ventricular fibrillation and sudden death. Based on the alterations in Ca^{2+}_i homeostasis discussed above, we investigated if the RV could play a defining role not only in the development of structural changes, but also in the occurrence of arrhythmias in the concealed early disease stage.[10,27] Taking a small step back in the timeline, we observed that RV CMs isolated at 14 DPI (hence, before structural changes) showed significantly increased amplitude and prolonged decay of Ca^{2+} transients when compared to CMs isolated from the LV. In addition, the frequency of Ca^{2+} sparks was significantly increased in the RV CMs from the mutant mouse hearts. Interestingly, this asymmetric behavior between RV and LV CMs was not observed in control CMs, suggesting that the differences in Ca^{2+} handling are directly correlated to PKP2 loss. Moreover, excessive Ca^{2+} accumulation was not only detected in the junctional sarcoplasmic reticulum, but also in the cytoplasmic and mitochondria compartments. It is also important to note that no transcriptional differences were observed at this time point. Rather, we detected functional changes likely resulting from events occurring after the transcriptional stage.

Increased Calcium Entry in the RV and the Role of Connexin43

Loss of gap junction plaques has been demonstrated in autoptic heart samples with ACM,[28] suggesting the existence of a currently well-accepted crosstalk of the different proteins residing at the intercalated disc. Further studies in cellular systems also showed that loss of PKP2 led to a redistribution of connexin43 (Cx43) inside the cells and reduced dye transfer between cells.[29] The subcellular localization or the abundance of Cx43 is not altered by the loss of PKP2 in the PKP2-cKO CMs. However, PKP2-cKO RV CMs demonstrated increased membrane permeability to Lucifer yellow dye-transfer; the latter could explain the excess Ca^{2+} detected in different compartments as being linked to an excessive availability of Cx43 hemichannels (Cx43-Hs).[27] An abnormal abundance of "orphan" Cx43-Hs can be consequent to altered intercellular adhesion, secondary to loss of PKP2 function,

which impairs proper gap junction formation. The increased Cx43-Hs abundance could be seen as one of the earliest manifestations of loss of PKP2 expression before macroscopic changes modify the structure and distribution of gap junctions (**Figure 3.2**). Interestingly, the asymmetrical difference in permeability between RV and LV myocytes was only detected in the very early stages of PKP2 loss, while both ventricles presented abnormally increased membrane permeability compared to controls a week after, which correspond to the 21 DPI timeline, where initial preclinical involvement of the LV is occurring. This result supports the progressive nature of molecular alterations typical of the ACM phenotype, and reinforce the role of altered Cx43-Hs abundance and Ca^{2+} homeostasis disruption in the different disease stages.

Functionally, we were able to correlate the increased Cx43-Hs availability to altered Ca^{2+} homeostasis by crossing the PKP2-cKO mouse with a cardiac-restricted heterozygous-null Cx43. This PKP2-cKO/Cx43+/− showed decreased Ca^{2+} sparks frequency compared to PKP2-cKO RV myocytes (**Figure 3.3**). Furthermore, selective Cx43-Hs inhibition by the TAT-Gap19 peptide blunted the effect of PKP2 loss in the RV in terms of Ca^{2+}_i disruption: indeed, sarcoplasmic reticulum load and Ca^{2+} transient amplitude were comparable to LV PKP2-cKO and to control myocytes in TAT-Gap19–treated RV myocytes.

Connexin43 Hemichannels and Fibrosis Progression

Interestingly, the contribution of Cx43 hemichannels to the ACM phenotype is not only restricted to facilitating arrhythmias at the molecular level but could also play a role in the progression of the fibrotic phenotype. In HL1 cells with RNA_i-mediated *PKP2* silencing, we observed an increase in ATP release provoked through a shift in osmotic pressure,

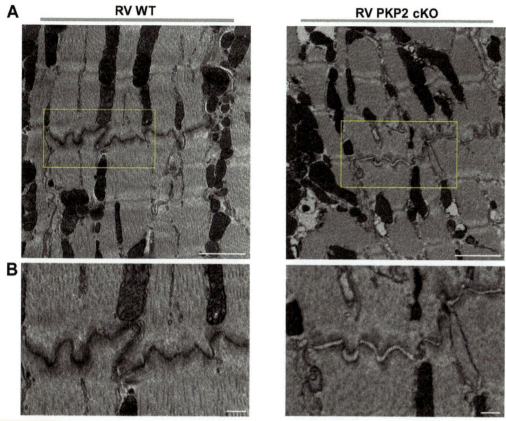

A   RV WT   RV PKP2 cKO

B

FIGURE 3.2   **Panel A:** Single frame of a complete FIB-SEM acquired set shows the ultrastructure of the intercalated disc from a control (**left**) and PKP2-cKO (**right**) RV sample. **Panel B:** Enlarged images from boxed yellow areas above come from the same tissue samples. Scale bars are 0.5 mm. There is evidence of increased intercellular distance in the sample from the PKP2-cKO heart. (Reproduced with permission from Kim et al., *Circulation*. 2019;140:1015–1030.[27])

a technique validated by other groups.[30] The possible opening of a hydrophilic pathway facilitating ATP release could be mediated by Cx43-H availability. Hence, we then used the same cell system, with a double knockout of both PKP2 and Cx43. As expected, absence of Cx43 availability blunted the excess adenosine triphosphate (ATP) release seen in the presence of PKP2 haploinsufficiency alone. In addition to this evidence, transcripts known to be part of the adenosine receptor cascade were overrepresented in our transcriptomic analysis of the PKP2-cKO murine hearts. Considering that ATP in the heart is rapidly converted to adenosine and that the role of different adenosine receptors has been involved in the progression of inflammation

and/or fibrosis in different organs, we treated PKP2-cKO hearts with a selective adenosine A2A receptor blocker, istradefylline, which is a drug approved in the market in the therapy of Parkinson's disease.[31] The mice received treatment for 3 weeks starting at 14 DPI, before the onset of structural damage. Histology analysis of end-stage hearts (35 DPI) revealed a significant decrease of collagen abundance in the RV and a tendency toward reduction in the LV, suggesting that blocking A2A adenosine receptors could limit or delay nonmyocytes cell recruitment in the interstitial space. Overall, it is possible to speculate that an excessive availability of Cx43-Hs in the setting of PKP2 loss could facilitate ATP release, which increases the activation of A2A

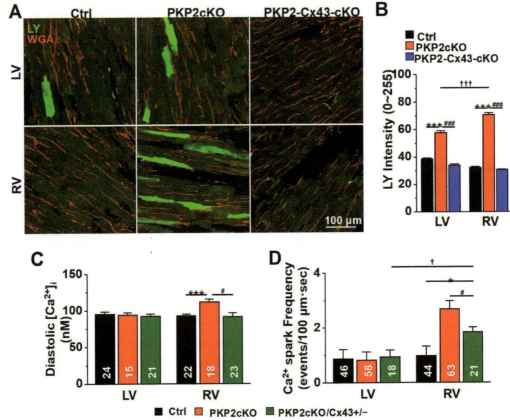

FIGURE 3.3 **Panel A:** Confocal images collected from the epicardial phase of either the LV or the RV free wall of hearts harvested from control (Ctrl), PKP2-cKO mice 14 DPI, or a double knockout of PKP2 and Cx43, also at 14 DPI (PKP2-Cx43-cKO). Images were obtained after a 30-min perfusion with 1 mg/mL Lucifer Yellow (LY; MW 457; **green**), 1 mg/mL Rhodamine Dextran (MW ~10,000), and 0.04 mg/mL Wheat Germ Agglutinin (WGA; **red**). **Panel B:** Average LY intensity was measured from cells in the following groups: Control (Ctrl; **black bars**), PKP2-cKO (**red bars**), and PKP2-Cx43-cKO (**blue bars**). ***$P <$ 0.001 vs. control; †††$P < 0.001$ vs. LV; ###$P < 0.001$ vs. PKP2-cKO. **Panel C:** Mean of the calculated values of $[Ca^{2+}]i$ after calibration of intensity ratios. PKP2-cKO/Cx43+/– refers to a PKP2-cKO mice also heterozygous-null for Cx43 in CMs. *$P < 0.05$ vs. control; #$P < 0.05$ vs. PKP2-cKO. **Panel D:** Ca^{2+} spark frequency is significantly dampened by reduced Cx43 expression (**green bar**). *$P < 0.05$ vs. control; †$P < 0.05$ vs. LV; PKP2-cKO. (Reproduced with permission from Kim et al., *Circulation*. 2019;140:1015–1030.[27])

PKP2-Dependent Transcription Network and Its Implications for Clinical ACM

As emphasized in the previous sections of this chapter, animal and cellular models have limitations, and often it is difficult to ascertain

adenosine receptors, and this could be one of the several intracellular signaling cascades participating in the fibrosis formation process.

the translational applicability of basic science findings into the human ACM phenotype. Transcriptomic studies are especially limited by the lack of availability of human affected hearts suitable for RNA extraction and handling. The recent availability of the GTex human repository,[32] which gathers transcriptome data from LV tissue derived from 272 heart donors, allowed us to compare experimental transcriptomic data against this human dataset. Although the human GTex data are not derived from affected patients, it is still possible to correlate a gene of choice, such as *PKP2*, with any other transcript of interest. Hence, it is possible to investigate if decreased *PKP2* transcript abundance correlates with decreased abundance of any other gene. This analysis revealed a good correlation between downregulated genes in the PKP2-cKO mouse and in the human GTex dataset.[11] Remarkably, pivotal genes involved in Ca^{2+} homeostasis, such as *RyR2, ANK2*, and *CACNA1c*, were significantly correlated with *PKP2* with extremely low false discovery rates (**Figure 3.4**).

Interestingly, expanding this correlation and analysis to the exploration of transcription factors that could be involved in the regulation of several of the downregulated genes, it was found that three transcription factors downregulated in the mouse model are also directly correlated with PKP2 in the human data. Not only did these transcription factors common to the two datasets control genes controlled them within the Ca^{2+} regulatory pathways, but they also controlled them within the fatty acid metabolism, a pathway identified not only in the PKP2-cKO mouse, but also in human ACM iPS-derived CMs.[11,33]

In a recent study, Wang et al.[34] corroborated the relation between desmosomal mutations and Ca^{2+} dysregulation. Their findings, though, pointed to integrin β1D as the link between the intercalated disc and the control of Ca^{2+} homeostasis.[34] Furthermore, the authors observed that desmosomal deficiency can lead to a PKA-mediated change in the phosphorylation state of RyR2 at Serine 2030. This is partly consistent with the results of Kim et al., who identified a new site in RyR2 (Thr 2809) only phosphorylated in RV myocytes following loss of *PKP2* expression.[27] Though these reports note different RyR2 sites (and likely different kinases), the data converge in indicating that desmosomal deficiency can disrupt the activity of RyR2 by kinase-mediated events. In broader terms, it also suggests that kinase derangement, likely caused (at least in part) by dislocation of intercalated disc-bound kinases after loss of desmosomal integrity, can phosphorylate (and affect the function of) multiple targets, giving way to the pleiotropic manifestations associated with desmosomal deficiency (Figure 3.4). Kinases may be the transducers of the intercalated disc transcription coupling reported in various models of ARVC.

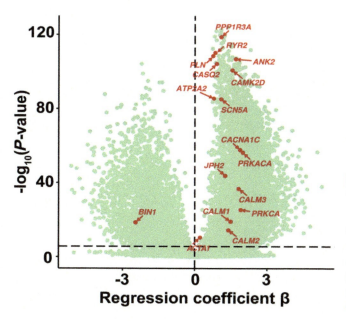

FIGURE 3.4 Association analysis of the human LV transcriptome in relation to PKP2 expression, with highlighted in **red** specific transcripts coding for proteins involved in intracellular calcium regulation. (Reproduced with permission from Montnach et al., *Europace*. 2018;20:iii125–iii132.[11])

Overall, the data indicate the existence of a molecular "axis" that links the intercalated disc to the regulation of Ca^{2+} release (**Figure 3.5**). Likely, this axis is coupled not by a single molecule but by multiple interconnected elements. Insofar, both Cx43-Hs27 and integrin β1D seem to be capable of connecting these two subcellular nanodomains (the intercalated disc on one hand; the dyad on the other) to affect function. A direct interaction between Cx43-Hs and RyR2 has also been demonstrated.[35] Both, Cx43-Hs and RyR2 channels represent attractive new targets for therapy. Regarding Cx43, it is important to emphasize that Cx43-Hs are not simply "half gap junctions." In fact, so far, molecules such as αCT-1,[36] RRNYRRNY,[37,38] or GAP19[39] that block Cx43-Hs do not block gap junction channels.

Furthermore, Cx43-Hs in ventricular myocytes seem to only open with increased probability when in a pathological state. As such, inhibitors of Cx43-Hs could, under pathological conditions, close a channel promoting arrhythmogenesis while not affecting the ability of cells to electrically couple to maintain propagation. With regard to RyR2, the Knollmann lab recently demonstrated that new, selective RyR2 blockers can blunt spontaneous RyR2-mediated Ca^{2+} release and effectively prevent arrhythmogenesis in an experimental model of CPVT characterized by excessive RyR2 eagerness to release Ca^{2+}.[40] Whether these or other compounds with similar effects can prove effective in experimental models, and as such advance toward clinical application, remains to be determined. There is, though, reasonable cause for cautious optimism.

Conclusions

The availability of multiple experimental systems and datasets, from cells, to animal models, to human data, has provided recently an increased body of evidence that the genetic substrate of ACM is linked to changes in genes or gene products whose functions transcend that of cell–cell adhesion. Our research has focused on loss of PKP2 and its spectrum of consequences, revealing that PKP2 has

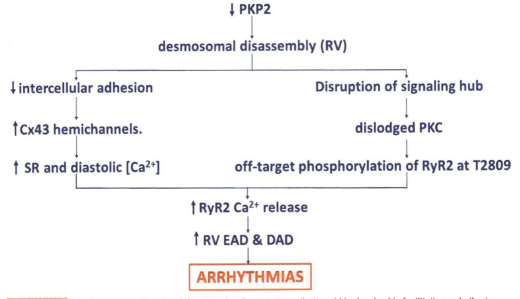

FIGURE 3.5 Flowchart summarizes the different molecular processes that could be involved in facilitating arrhythmias in the PKP2-cKO mouse hearts. Abbreviations: Cx43, connexin43; DAD, delayed after-depolarization; EAD, early after-depolarization; PKC, phosphokinase C; RV, right ventricle; SR, sarcoplasmic reticulum.

several different roles aside from the preservation of desmosomal integrity. Its localization at the intercalated disc could affect proper membrane trafficking of ion channels and other proteins. In addition, several data support the notion that PKP2 is part of a coordinated network of transcripts that include proteins of the mechanical junctions, regulators of cell metabolism, and proteins that control cardiac intracellular calcium levels. Overall, the acknowledgment that a gene and a protein have a wider pleiotropic realm of functions than the one initially attributed upon their discovery opens a new perspective in the study of the molecular mechanisms of inherited arrhythmogenic diseases, with ACM being one of the earliest conditions that has been investigated under this more current perspective. This novel integrative approach could also provide a novel viewpoint in the investigation of the mechanisms underlying the different disease aspects and offer new targets for therapeutic approaches, which are still insufficient in controlling ACM lethality and disease progression.

References

1. Corrado D, Link MS, Calkins H. Arrhythmogenic right ventricular cardiomyopathy. *N Engl J Med*. 2017;376:61–72.

2. Basso C, Corrado D, Marcus FI, Nava A, Thiene G. Arrhythmogenic right ventricular cardiomyopathy. *Lancet*. 2009;373:1289–300.

3. Philips B, Cheng A. 2015 update on the diagnosis and management of arrhythmogenic right ventricular cardiomyopathy. *Curr Opin Cardiol*. 2016;31:46–56.

4. Groeneweg JA, Bhonsale A, James CA, et al. Clinical presentation, long-term follow-up, and outcomes of 1001 arrhythmogenic right ventricular dysplasia/cardiomyopathy patients and family members. *Circ Cardiovasc Genet*. 2015;8:437–446.

5. James CA, Bhonsale A, Tichnell C, et al. Exercise increases age-related penetrance and arrhythmic risk in arrhythmogenic right

6. Bhonsale A, Groeneweg JA, James CA, et al. Impact of genotype on clinical course in arrhythmogenic right ventricular dysplasia/cardiomyopathy-associated mutation carriers. *Eur Heart J*. 2015;36:847–855.

7. Lazzarini E, Jongbloed JD, Pilichou K, et al. The ARVD/C genetic variants database: 2014 update. *Human Mut*. 2015;36:403–410.

8. Kant S, Holthofer B, Magin TM, Krusche CA, Leube RE. Desmoglein 2-dependent arrhythmogenic cardiomyopathy is caused by a loss of adhesive function. *Circ Cardiovasc Genet*. 2015;8:553–563.

9. Yang Z, Bowles NE, Scherer SE, et al. Desmosomal dysfunction due to mutations in desmoplakin causes arrhythmogenic right ventricular dysplasia/cardiomyopathy. *Circ Res*. 2006;99:646–555.

10. Cerrone M, Montnach J, Lin X, et al. Plakophilin-2 is required for transcription of genes that control calcium cycling and cardiac rhythm. *Nat Commun*. 2017;8:106.

11. Montnach J, Agullo-Pascual E, Tadros R, Bezzina CR, Delmar M. Bioinformatic analysis of a plakophilin-2-dependent transcription network: Implications for the mechanisms of arrhythmogenic right ventricular cardiomyopathy in humans and in boxer dogs. *Europace*. 2018;20:iii125–iii132.

12. Dubash AD, Kam CY, Aguado BA, et al. Plakophilin-2 loss promotes TGF-beta1/p38 MAPK-dependent fibrotic gene expression in cardiomyocytes. *J Cell Biol*. 2016;212:425–438.

13. Grossmann KS, Grund C, Huelsken J, et al. Requirement of plakophilin 2 for heart morphogenesis and cardiac junction formation. *J Cell Biol*. 2004;167:149–160.

14. van Opbergen CJM, Noorman M, Pfenniger A, et al. Plakophilin-2 haploinsufficiency causes calcium handling deficits and modulates the cardiac response towards stress. *Int J Mol Sci*. 2019;20:4076.

15. Cerrone M, Noorman M, Lin X, et al. Sodium current deficit and arrhythmogenesis in a

murine model of plakophilin-2 haploinsufficiency. *Cardiovasc Res.* 2012;95:460–468.

16. Agullo-Pascual E, Cerrone M, Delmar M. Arrhythmogenic cardiomyopathy and Brugada syndrome: Diseases of the connexome. *FEBS Lett.* 2014;588:1322–1330.

17. Agullo-Pascual E, Reid DA, Keegan S, Sidhu M, Fenyo D, Rothenberg E, Delmar M. Super-resolution fluorescence microscopy of the cardiac connexome reveals plakophilin-2 inside the connexin43 plaque. *Cardiovasc Res.* 2013;100:231–240.

18. Leo-Macias A, Liang FX, Delmar M. Ultrastructure of the intercellular space in adult murine ventricle revealed by quantitative tomographic electron microscopy. *Cardiovasc Res.* 2015;107:442–452.

19. Che SN, Gurha P, Lombardi R, Ruggiero A, Willerson JT, Marian AJ. The hippo pathway is activated and is a causal mechanism for adipogenesis in arrhythmogenic cardiomyopathy. *Circ Res.* 2014;114:454–468.

20. van der Werf C, Kannankeril PJ, Sacher F, et al. Flecainide therapy reduces exercise-induced ventricular arrhythmias in patients with catecholaminergic polymorphic ventricular tachycardia. *J Am Coll Cardiol.* 2011;57:2244–254.

21. Itzhaki I, Maizels L, Huber I, et al. Modeling of catecholaminergic polymorphic ventricular tachycardia with patient-specific human-induced pluripotent stem cells. *J Am Coll Cardiol.* 2012;60:990–1000.

22. Hwang HS, Hasdemir C, Laver D, et al. Inhibition of cardiac Ca2+ release channels (RyR2) determines efficacy of class I antiarrhythmic drugs in catecholaminergic polymorphic ventricular tachycardia. *Circ Arrhythm Electrophysiol.* 2011;4:128–135.

23. Watanabe H, van der Werf C, Roses-Noguer F, et al. Effects of flecainide on exercise-induced ventricular arrhythmias and recurrences in genotype-negative patients with catecholaminergic polymorphic ventricular tachycardia. *Heart Rhythm.* 2013;10:542–547.

24. Kannankeril PJ, Moore JP, Cerrone M, et al. Efficacy of flecainide in the treatment of catecholaminergic polymorphic ventricular tachycardia: A randomized clinical trial. *JAMA Cardiol.* 2017;2:759–766.

25. Tester DJ, Ackerman JP, Giudicessi JR, Ackerman NC, Cerrone M, Delmar M, Ackerman MJ. Plakophilin-2 truncation variants in patients clinically diagnosed with catecholaminergic polymorphic ventricular tachycardia and decedents with exercise-associated autopsy negative sudden unexplained death in the young. *JACC Clin Electrophysiol.* 2019;5:120–127.

26. Ermakov S, Gerstenfeld EP, Svetlichnaya Y, Scheinman MM. Use of flecainide in combination antiarrhythmic therapy in patients with arrhythmogenic right ventricular cardiomyopathy. *Heart Rhythm.* 2017;14:564–569.

27. Kim JC, Perez-Hernandez Duran M, Alvarado FJ, et al. Disruption of Ca(2+)i homeostasis and Cx43 hemichannel function in the right ventricle precedes overt arrhythmogenic cardiomyopathy in PKP2-deficient mice. *Circulation.* 2019;140:1015–1030.

28. Noorman M, Hakim S, Kessler E, et al. Remodeling of the cardiac sodium channel, connexin43, and plakoglobin at the intercalated disk in patients with arrhythmogenic cardiomyopathy. *Heart Rhythm.* 2013;10:412–419.

29. Oxford EM, Musa H, Maass K, Coombs W, Taffet SM, Delmar M. Connexin43 remodeling caused by inhibition of plakophilin-2 expression in cardiac cells. *Circ Res.* 2007;101:703–711.

30. Cerrone M, van Opbergen CJM, Malkani K, et al. Blockade of the adenosine 2A receptor mitigates the cardiomyopathy induced by loss of plakophilin-2 expression. *Front Physiol.* 2018;9:1750.

31. Muller T. The safety of istradefylline for the treatment of Parkinson's disease. *Expert Opin Drug Saf.* 2015;14:769–775.

32. Veerman CC, Podliesna S, Tadros R, et al. The Brugada syndrome susceptibility gene HEY2 modulates cardiac transmural ion channel patterning and electrical heterogeneity. *Circ Res.* 2017;121:537–548.

33. Kim C, Wong J, Wen J, et al. Studying arrhythmogenic right ventricular dysplasia

with patient-specific iPSCs. *Nature.* 2013;494:105–110.

34. Wang Y LC, Shi L, Chen X, et al. Integrin 1 β1D deficiency-mediated RyR2 dysfunction contributes to catecholamine-sensitive ventricular tachycardia in ARVC. *Circulation.* 2020;141:1477–1493.

35. Lissoni A, Hulpiau P, Martins-Marques T, et al. RyR2 regulates Cx43 hemichannel intracellular Ca2+-dependent activation in cardiomyocytes. *Cardiovasc Res.* 2019 Dec 16;cvz340. doi: 10.1093/cvr/cvz340. Online ahead of print.

36. Jiang J, Hoagland D, Palatinus JA, et al. Interaction of alpha carboxyl terminus 1 peptide with the connexin 43 carboxyl terminus preserves left ventricular function after ischemia-reperfusion injury. *J Am Heart Assoc.* 2019;8:e012385.

37. Verma V, Larsen BD, Coombs W, et al. Novel pharmacophores of connexin43 based on the "RXP" series of Cx43-binding peptides. *Circ Res.* 2009;105:176–184.

38. Gadicherla AK, Wang N, Bulic M, et al. Mitochondrial Cx43 hemichannels contribute to mitochondrial calcium entry and cell death in the heart. *Basic Res Cardiol.* 2017;112:27.

39. Wang N, De Vuyst E, Ponsaerts R, et al. Selective inhibition of Cx43 hemichannels by Gap19 and its impact on myocardial ischemia/reperfusion injury. *Basic Res Cardiol.* 2013;108:309.

40. Batiste SM, Blackwell DJ, Kim K, et al. Unnatural verticilide enantiomer inhibits type 2 ryanodine receptor-mediated calcium leak and is antiarrhythmic. *Proc Natl Acad Sci USA.* 2019;116:4810–4815.

4

Immune Signaling in Arrhythmogenic Cardiomyopathy

Stephen P. Chelko, PhD; Angeliki Asimaki, PhD; Justin Lowenthal, BS; Carlos Bueno-Beti, PhD; Alexandros Protonotarios, MD; Leslie Tung, PhD; Jeffrey E. Saffitz, MD, PhD

Introduction

Myocardial inflammation is often prominent in arrhythmogenic cardiomyopathy (ACM). Inflammatory infiltrates occur in the hearts of 60% to 88% of ACM patients, and are especially common in ACM patients who died suddenly.[1–3] They typically involve both ventricles even if macroscopic disease is confined to the right ventricle (RV).[3] A histologic picture reminiscent of acute myocarditis may be associated with an active phase of ACM characterized by accelerated disease progression.[4] In addition, ACM patients exhibit elevated circulating levels of proinflammatory cytokines, and cardiac myocytes themselves produce potent cytokines in ACM.[5] Thus, inflammation in ACM involves infiltrating inflammatory cells *and* apparent activation of an innate immune response in cardiac myocytes. However, the role of inflammation as a driver of the ACM disease phenotype has not been studied previously.

Nuclear factor κB (NFκB) is a master regulator of cellular inflammatory responses initiated by diverse injurious agents including stress, proinflammatory cytokines, reactive oxygen species, heavy metals, UV radiation, oxidized LDL, and bacterial/viral antigens.[6,7] It is found in virtually all animal cells including cardiac myocytes. Accordingly, we have recently explored the role of inflammatory signaling mediated by NFκB in promoting myocardial damage, contractile dysfunction, and cytokine production in ACM. Our work shows that NFκB signaling is, indeed, activated in ACM.[8] Moreover, blocking inflammatory signaling with a small-molecule inhibitor of NFκB shows a remarkable ability to rescue the disease phenotype in ACM models in vitro and *in vivo* involving expression of three different alleles known to cause disease in patients.[8] Thus, inflammation is a driver of arrhythmias and myocardial injury in ACM.

Inhibition of NFκB Signaling Reverses ACM Disease Features *In Vitro*

We first characterized inflammatory signaling in primary cultures of neonatal rat ventricular myocytes transfected to express a disease causing allele of the desmosomal protein plakoglobin ($JUP^{2157del2}$).[9] These cells exhibit several features in vitro that occur in the hearts of ACM patients, including redistribution of plakoglobin (also known as γ-catenin) from cell–cell junctions into the cytosol and nucleus; loss of cell-surface immunoreactive signal for the major cardiac gap junction protein, connexin43 (Cx43); redistribution of GSK3β from the cytosol to the cell surface; and myocyte apoptosis.[9,10] We found that immunoreactive signal for phospho-RelA/p65 (Ser536) accumulates in the nuclei of cardiac myocytes expressing $JUP^{2157del2}$, indicating activation of NFκB signaling in this in vitro model of ACM. Treatment of these cells with Bay 11-7082, a small-molecule inhibitor of NFκB signaling, prevented nuclear accumulation of phospho-RelA/p65 (**Figure 4.1**, Panel A).[8] It also diminished expression and secretion of proinflammatory cytokines (Figure 4.1, Panel B), and normalized the aberrant distribution of key proteins including plakoglobin, Cx43, and GSK3β (Figure 4.1, Panel C).[8] Finally, myocyte apoptosis, measured by TUNEL labeling, was increased by roughly 10-fold in ACM myocytes but returned to control levels in cells exposed to Bay 11-7082 for 24 hours (Figure 4.1, Panels D and E).[8]

Inhibition of NFκB Signaling Prevents Development of ACM Disease Features *In Vivo*

We next characterized NFκB signaling *in vivo* in a mouse model of ACM involving homozygous knockin of a mutant form of *Dsg2*, the gene encoding the desmosomal cadherin desmoglein-2 ($Dsg2^{mut/mut}$ mice).[10] The mutation entails loss of exons 4 and 5, which causes a frameshift and premature termination of translation. As reported previously, $Dsg2^{mut/mut}$ mice show no cardiac structural or functional derangements at 8 weeks of age, but during the ensuing 8 weeks, they develop electrocardiogram (ECG) changes and progressive contractile dysfunction associated with myocardial necrosis, fibrosis, and inflammation.[10] These structural and functional changes are accompanied by marked shifts in the distribution of various cardiac myocyte proteins including desmosomal proteins, connexins and ion channel proteins, proteins involved in the Wnt/β-catenin signaling pathway, and synapse-associated protein 97 (SAP97), a chaperone protein involved in ion channel transport to intercalated disks.[10]

To determine if NFκB pathways are activated in the hearts of $Dsg2^{mut/mut}$ mice at 16 weeks of age, we performed Western blots to measure levels of total RelA/p65 and phospho-RelA/p65 (Ser536) in myocardial homogenates. As shown in **Figure 4.2**, Panels A and B, the amount of total myocardial RelA/p65 was equivalent in control (wildtype) and $Dsg2^{mut/mut}$ mice, but phospho-RelA/p65 was significantly increased in the hearts of $Dsg2^{mut/mut}$ mice.[8] Treatment of $Dsg2^{mut/mut}$ mice with Bay 11-7082 reduced the amount of phospho-RelA/p65 to levels equivalent to that seen in control hearts, thus showing that NFκB is activated in the hearts of $Dsg2^{mut/mut}$ mice and Bay 11-7082 is sufficient to block this signaling pathway.[8]

Next, to determine if inhibition of inflammatory signaling mitigates development of the ACM phenotype *in vivo*, we treated $Dsg2^{mut/mut}$ mice with Bay 11-7082 by continuous infusion over an 8-week period beginning when the mice were 8 weeks of age. As shown in Figure 4.2, Panels C–J, treatment of $Dsg2^{mut/mut}$ mice with Bay 11-7082 normalized contractile function and significantly reduced the amount of

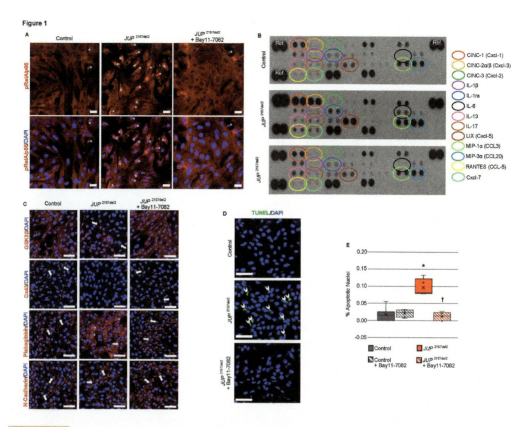

FIGURE 4.1 Activation of NFκB and reversal of ACM features by Bay 11-7082 in neonatal rat ventricular myocytes (NRVMs) expressing a deletion mutation in the gene encoding plakoglobin (*JUP*[2157del2]). **Panel A:** Phospho-RelA/p65 (pRelA/p65) is shown as red signal in representative confocal immunofluorescence images from control (nontransfected) NRVMs and NRVMs expressing *JUP*[2157del2] in the absence or presence of Bay 11-7082. Nuclear accumulation of immunoreactive signal, indicating activation of NFκB, is readily apparent in cells expressing *JUP*[2157del2] (**asterisks**) but is absent in such cells after treatment with Bay 11-7082. Scale bar = 50 μm. **Panel B:** Representative cytokine arrays prepared from culture media from control (nontransfected) cells and NRVMs expressing *JUP*[2157del2] in the absence or presence of Bay 11-7082. The spots in the **upper right** and left and **lower left corners** are reference markers (Ref Bands) to compare overall exposure levels. **Panel C:** Distribution of selected cell–cell junction and signaling proteins in representative confocal immunofluorescence images from control (nontransfected) NRVMs and NRVMs expressing *JUP*[2157del2] in the absence or presence of Bay 11-7082. **Arrows** show localization of immunoreactive signal at the cell surface. The normal distribution of N-cadherin in all cells is shown as a positive control. Untreated *JUP*[2157del2] cells showed abnormal distribution of plakoglobin, Cx43, and GSK3β. The amount of signal for plakoglobin and Cx43 at cell–cell junctions was greatly reduced in these cells whereas signal for GSK3β, which normally resides in the cytoplasm, was seen at the cell surface. **Asterisks** identify apparent nuclear localization of plakoglobin in *JUP*[2157del2] cells. The abnormal distribution of plakoglobin, Cx43 and GSK3β was normalized in *JUP*[2157del2] cells treated with Bay 11-7082. Scale bar = 50 μm. **Panel D:** TUNEL + nuclei (**arrow heads**) in control NRVMs and NRVMs expressing *JUP*[2157del2] in the absence or presence of Bay 11-7082. Scale bar = 50 μm. **Panel E:** Graph shows the percent (%) apoptotic nuclei in 5 microscopic fields from each condition. * $P < 0.0001$ for *JUP*[2157del2] cells vs. control cells and †$P < 0.0001$ for Bay 11-7082-treated vs. untreated *JUP*[2157del2] cells determined by one-way analysis of variance (ANOVA) with Tukey's multiple comparisons test.

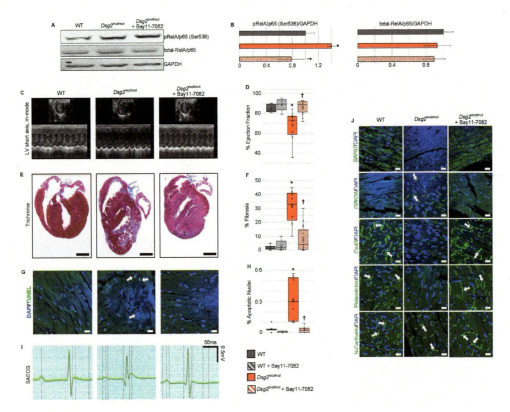

FIGURE 4.2 Activation of NFκB and reversal of ACM disease features in Dsg2$^{mut/mut}$ mice *in vivo* by inhibition of NFκB signaling with Bay 11-7082. **Panel A:** Western blots of total RelA/p65 and phospho-RelA/p65 in homogenates of hearts from vehicle-treated wildtype (WT) mice, and vehicle- and Bay 11-7082-treated Dsg2$^{mut/mut}$ mice. **Panel B:** Group data for total-RelA/p65 and pRelA/p65 (Ser536) protein levels in hearts of vehicle-treated WT mice, and vehicle- and Bay 11-7082-treated Dsg2$^{mut/mut}$ mice. **Panel C:** Representative short-axis m-mode ECGs of vehicle-treated wildtype (WT) mice, Dsg2$^{mut/mut}$ mice and Dsg2$^{mut/mut}$ mice treated with Bay 11-7082. **Panel D:** Group data for percent ejection fraction in vehicle- and Bay 11-7082-treated wildtype (WT) mice, and vehicle- and Bay 11-7082-treated Dsg2$^{mut/mut}$ mice. **Panel E:** Representative long-axis sections of the hearts stained with Masson trichrome from wildtype (WT) mice, Dsg2$^{mut/mut}$ mice, and Dsg2$^{mut/mut}$ mice treated with Bay 11-7082. Scale bar = 1 mm. **Panel F:** Group data for percentage of LV area occupied by fibrosis in Masson trichrome-stained sections of hearts from vehicle- and Bay 11-7082-treated wildtype (WT) mice, and vehicle- and Bay 11-7082-treated Dsg2$^{mut/mut}$ mice. **Panel G:** Representative images show TUNEL labeling in sections of hearts from wildtype (WT) mice, Dsg2$^{mut/mut}$ mice, and Dsg2$^{mut/mut}$ mice treated with Bay 11-7082. **Arrows** show TUNEL+ nuclei. Scale bar = 10 μm. **Panel H:** Group data show percentage of apoptotic nuclei in TUNEL-labeled sections of hearts from vehicle- and Bay 11-7082-treated wildtype (WT) mice, and vehicle- and Bay 11-7082-treated Dsg2$^{mut/mut}$ mice. **Panel I:** Representative signal-averaged electrocardiograms (SAECGs) from WT mice, Dsg2$^{mut/mut}$ mice, and Dsg2$^{mut/mut}$ mice treated with Bay 11-7082. **Panel J:** Representative confocal images of immunostained hearts from wildtype (WT) mice, Dsg2$^{mut/mut}$ mice, and Dsg2$^{mut/mut}$ mice treated with Bay 11-7082. **Arrows** show localization of immunoreactive signal at the cell surface. The normal distribution of N-cadherin in all cohorts is shown as a positive control. Untreated Dsg2$^{mut/mut}$ mice showed abnormal distribution of plakoglobin, Cx43, GSK3β, and SAP97. The amount of signal for plakoglobin, Cx43, and SAP97 at cell–cell junctions was greatly reduced, whereas signal for GSK3β, which normally resides in the cytoplasm, was seen at the cell surface. These abnormal protein distributions were normalized in Dsg2$^{mut/mut}$ mice treated with Bay 11-7082. Scale bar = 10 μm. Quantitative data in Panels B, D, F, and H are shown as mean ± SEM; n = 10 for vehicle-treated WT mice; n = 5 for Bay 11-7082-treated WT mice; n = 9 for vehicle-treated Dsg2$^{mut/mut}$ mice; and n = 17 for Bay 11-7082-treated Dsg2$^{mut/mut}$ mice. *$P < 0.001$ for vehicle-treated Dsg2$^{mut/mut}$ mice vs. vehicle-treated WT mice; and †$P < 0.001$ for Bay 11-7082-treated Dsg2$^{mut/mut}$ mice vs. vehicle-treated Dsg2$^{mut/mut}$ mice as determined by one-way ANOVA with Tukey's multiple comparisons test.

ventricular necrosis, apoptosis, and fibrosis.[8] It also corrected abnormalities in the SAECG. Finally, Bay 11-7082-treated mice showed no apparent derangements in the distributions of plakoglobin, Cx43, GSK3β, and SAP97.[8]

The Heart Contains Abundant Cytokines in ACM

Activation of NFκB pathways in the hearts of $Dsg2^{mut/mut}$ mice likely stimulates expression of inflammatory mediators. To characterize production of chemical mediators of the immune response in ACM, we used arrays to measure cytokines in the hearts of $Dsg2^{mut/mut}$ mice and compared the amounts to levels in the hearts of WT mice and $Dsg2^{mut/mut}$ mice treated with Bay 11-7082. **Figure 4.3** shows data for selected molecules including powerful proinflammatory cytokines such as IL-1β (up by ~13-fold compared to control hearts), IFNγ (~5-fold), IL-12 (~6-fold), and TNFα (~2-fold).[8] Expression of various chemotactic molecules was also greatly increased in $Dsg2^{mut/mut}$ hearts, including the B-cell chemoattractant CXCL13 (up by ~6-fold), M-CSF (~20-fold), and the neutrophil chemoattractant LIX (CXCL5; ~60-fold). And, expression of various pleomorphic molecules with multiple actions was also increased including HGF (~15-fold) and P-selectin (~40-fold). Finally, some molecules that fulfill anti-inflammatory roles such as IL-1Ra were also increased in $Dsg2^{mut/mut}$ hearts (by ~4-fold). To a varying degree, treatment with Bay 11-7082 reversed or at least blunted cytokine levels (Figure 4.3).[8]

Chemical mediators of the immune response are expressed both by the professional cells of the adaptive immune system (mainly lymphocytes and macrophages) and by parenchymal cells of many organs including the heart. To identify the cellular source of cytokines in $Dsg2^{mut/mut}$ mice, we stained sections of myocardium with antibodies against representative key molecules including IL-1β, TNFα, and MCP-1α. As shown in **Figure 4.4**, cardiac myocytes exhibited positive immunoreactive signal for IL-1β, TNFα, and MCP-1α, whereas positive signal for IL-1β and TNFα was seen in infiltrating mononuclear inflammatory cells that included both macrophages and T cells.[8] Thus, inflammation in ACM involves activation of an immune response on the part of infiltrating cells in cells and by cardiac myocytes driven, at least in part, by NFκB signaling.

ACM Patient hiPSC-Cardiac Myocytes Express Abundant Cytokines Under the Control of NFκB

To gain further insights into the immune response in ACM, we characterized immunoreactive signal for phospho-RelA/p65 (Ser536) and cytokine production in cultures of cardiac myocytes derived from hiPSC-cardiac myocytes (hiPSC-CMs) obtained from a patient with documented ACM caused by a mutation in the desmosomal gene PKP2.[9] These cultures contain more than 95% pure cardiac myocytes, and are devoid of lymphocytes and macrophages. As shown in **Figure 4.5**, when grown under basal conditions, these ACM patient cardiac myocytes displayed marked nuclear accumulation of phospho-RelA/p65 (Ser536) indicating activation of NFκB signaling pathways.[8] They also expressed and secreted into the culture medium large amounts of cytokines including essentially all that were expressed in the hearts of $Dsg2^{mut/mut}$ mice. Exposure of ACM patient hiPSC-CMs to Bay 11-7082 prevented nuclear accumulation of phospho-RelA/p65 and greatly reduced the amount of cytokines in cells and culture media (Figure 4.5).[8] These observations provide additional independent evidence of activation of an innate immune response in cardiac myocytes in ACM under the control of NFκB signaling.

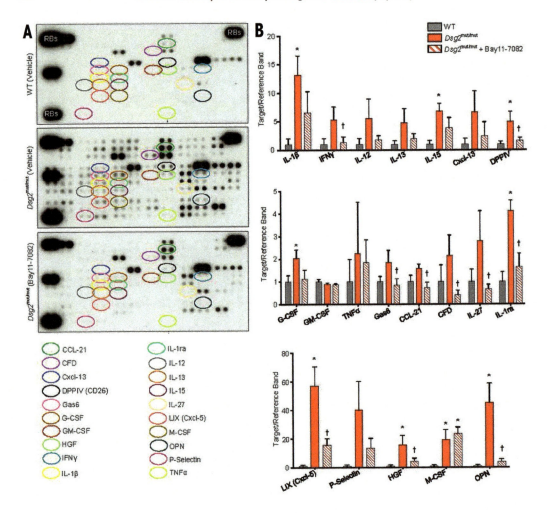

FIGURE 4.3 Cytokine expression in the hearts of Dsg2$^{mut/mut}$ mice and its attenuation by Bay 11-7082 are presented. **Panel A:** Representative cytokine arrays from myocardial lysates from vehicle-treated wildtype (WT) mice, Dsg2$^{mut/mut}$ mice, and Dsg2$^{mut/mut}$ mice treated with Bay 11-7082. The spots in the upper right and left and lower left corners are reference markers (RBs) to compare overall exposure levels. **Panel B:** Quantitative data for expression of selected cytokines in hearts of vehicle-treated WT mice, Dsg2$^{mut/mut}$ mice, and Dsg2$^{mut/mut}$ mice treated with Bay 11-7082. Data are shown as mean ± SEM; n = 5 for each cytokine in vehicle-treated WT and Dsg2$^{mut/mut}$ mice; and n = 10 for each cytokine in Bay11-7082-treated Dsg2$^{mut/mut}$ mice; *$P < 0.05$ for any cohort vs. vehicle-treated WT mice; and †$P < 0.05$ for Bay 11-7082-treated Dsg2$^{mut/mut}$ mice vs. vehicle-treated Dsg2$^{mut/mut}$ mice as determined by one-way ANOVA with Tukey's multiple comparisons test.

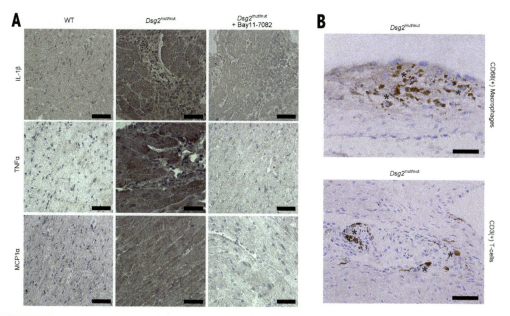

FIGURE 4.4 Cytokine expression in CMs and infiltrating inflammatory cells in hearts of Dsg2$^{mut/mut}$ mice. **Panel A:** Sections of myocardium are presented from vehicle-treated wildtype (WT) mice, Dsg2$^{mut/mut}$ mice, and Dsg2$^{mut/mut}$ mice treated with Bay 11-7082 showing immunoperoxidase signals for IL-1β, TNFα, and MCP1α. Signal intensities for all 3 cytokines were increased in myocardial sections from Dsg2$^{mut/mut}$ mice. Signals for IL-1β and TNFα were seen in both cardiac myocytes and infiltrating inflammatory cells in hearts of Dsg2$^{mut/mut}$ mice. Treatment with Bay 11-7082 reduced signal intensity. **Panel B:** Sections of myocardium from Dsg2$^{mut/mut}$ mice show immunoperoxidase signals for macrophages (CD68 + cells) and T cells (CD3 + cells) (asterisks). Scale bar = 25 μm.

Discussion

The ability of cells to produce immune mediators and recognition systems that respond to injury and distinguish self from nonself appeared approximately 600 million years ago.[11,12] Such innate immune mechanisms can be found in primitive invertebrates such as sponges and cnidarians.[11,12] They differ from the far more recent development of the adaptive (or acquired) immune response in vertebrates, which is highly specific for a given pathogen. The conventional view of myocardial inflammation involves infiltration of the heart by inflammatory cells and myocardial injury mediated by injurious molecules produced by such bone marrow derived cells. Nevertheless, heart failure due to various etiologies and types of injury such as ischemia/reperfusion or pressure overload is also associated with myocardial production of proinflammatory molecules of the innate immune response in the absence of conspicuous inflammatory cell infiltration.[13] Major cytokines in the failing heart include TNFα, IL-6, and IL-1β, which act as mediators of tissue injury.[13] For example, IL-6, produced by both cardiac myocytes and myeloid cells (neutrophils and macrophages), upregulates ICAM-1 on cardiac myocytes, which mediates neutrophil binding and promotes cytotoxic actions.[13] Myocardial inflammation thus entails a diverse array of innate and adaptive immune mechanisms involving activation of various signaling pathways that regulate, in a highly context-dependent fashion, cytokine production, inflammation, cell survival or death, and cell proliferation.

Here, we present evidence that the pathogenesis of ACM involves immune signaling. We found that NFκB is activated in three dif-

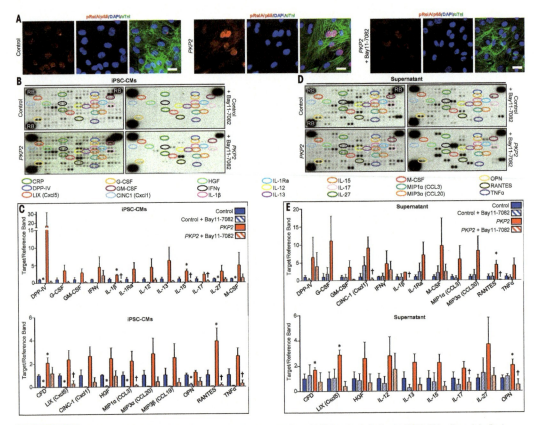

FIGURE 4.5 Activation of NFκB and cytokine expression in control and ACM patient-derived hiPSC-CMs. **Panel A:** Red immunoreactive signal for phospho-RelA/p65 (pRelA/p65) in confocal images from cultures of cardiac myocytes derived from a control hiPSC cell line and a line from an ACM patient with a pathogenic variant in plakophilin-2 (*PKP2*) grown in the absence or presence of Bay 11-7082. Virtually all *PKP2* cells are positive for cardiac troponin-I (cTnI), indicating they are cardiac myocytes. Control hiPSC-CMs showed normal prominent cell surface staining for plakoglobin. Marked nuclear accumulation of phospho-RelA/p65 is seen in *PKP2* hiPSC-CMs but not in control cells. Treatment of *PKP2* hiPSC-CMs with Bay 11-7082 prevented nuclear accumulation of phospho-RelA/p65 signal. Scale bar = 20 μm. **Panel B:** Representative cytokine arrays prepared from cultures of cardiac myocytes derived from a control hiPSC cell line and a line from a patient with a disease-causing variant in plakophillin-2 (*PKP2*). Arrays are shown for cells grown in the absence (untreated) or presence of Bay 11-7082. The **spots in the upper right and left and lower left corners** are reference markers (RBs) to compare overall exposure levels. **Panel C:** Quantitative data (mean ± SEM; n = 3 for each cohort and condition) for expression of selected cytokines in control and *PKP2* cells with or without Bay 11-7082. *$P < 0.05$ for any cohort vs. control cardiac myocytes; $^{†}P < 0.05$ for Bay 11-7082-treated *PKP2* cardiac myocytes vs. untreated *PKP2* cardiac myocytes. **Panel D:** Representative cytokine arrays prepared from culture media (supernatant) from cardiac myocytes derived from a control hiPSC cell line and a line from a patient with a disease-causing variant in *PKP2*. Arrays are shown for media isolated from cells grown in the absence or presence of Bay 11-7082. The **spots in the upper right and left and lower left corners** are reference markers (RBs) to compare overall exposure levels. **Panel E:** Quantitative data (mean ± SEM; n = 3 for each cohort and condition) for expression of selected cytokines in media from control and PKP2 cells with or without Bay 11-7082. *$P < 0.05$ for any cohort vs. control cardiac myocytes; $^{†}P < 0.05$ for Bay 11-7082-treated *PKP2* cardiac myocytes vs. untreated *PKP2* cardiac myocytes. Statistical analyses in **Panels C** and **E** were performed using one-way ANOVA with Tukey's multiple comparisons test.

ferent experimental models of ACM involving expression of three different desmosomal gene variants known to cause disease in patients. This was demonstrated by observing increased expression and/or nuclear accumulation of phospho-RelA/p65, which are hallmarks of activation of the NFκB signaling cascade.[6,7] Such changes in phospho-RelA/p65 were blocked by the small molecule Bay 11-7082, thus confirming that it acts to inhibit NFκB signaling. We also found that Bay 11-7082 has a remarkable ability to rescue ACM phenotypes in an in vitro model involving transfected primary cardiac myocytes and a robust mouse model *in vivo*. Finally, we showed that NFκB signaling is activated in cardiac myocytes derived from an ACM patient with a pathogenic variant in *PKP2*. These ACM patient cardiac myocytes produced and secreted large amounts of proinflammatory cytokines under basal conditions without the need for provocative stimuli. Taken together, these observations indicate that disease-causing variants in multiple desmosomal genes are sufficient to activate a cell autonomous immune response in cardiac myocytes. They also provide new insights into immune mechanisms in the pathogenesis of ACM and identify a potential new therapeutic approach to limit myocardial damage and reduce the risk of serious arrhythmias in patients.

The idea that NFκB signaling participates in the pathogenesis of ACM is strongly supported by "experiments of nature" involving naturally occurring variants in *Nkip1*, the gene that encodes NFκB interacting protein 1 (also known as *PPP1R13L*). For example, a deletion mutation in this gene has been linked to a spontaneous disorder in mice characterized by cardiomyopathy and abnormal skin.[14] Another mutation in the same gene has been identified in Poll Hereford cattle with a spontaneously occurring lethal syndrome of cardiomyopathy and woolly hair coat reminiscent of Naxos syndrome in patients.[15,16]

Nkip1, expressed in skin, heart, and vascular endothelium, is a member of a small family of transcriptional regulators. A C-terminal fragment of *Nkip1* has been shown to be a RelA associated inhibitor.[14] Thus, loss of function mutations might be expected to constitutively activate NFκB signaling in tissues in which the gene is expressed.

The immune response in ACM has two components, both of which likely contribute to disease pathogenesis. The first component, infiltration of the myocardium by "professional" cells of the adaptive immune response (lymphocytes and macrophages), is the most conspicuous. Indeed, inflammatory cells can be so abundant in the hearts of ACM patients that the disease may be misdiagnosed as myocarditis.[17] However, it has never been clear if inflammatory cells accumulate in the heart in ACM only as a reparative response to myocardial damage or if such cells actually promote arrhythmias and/or myocyte injury mediated by immune mechanisms. The second component involves activation of an innate immune response in cardiac myocytes in ACM. How this occurs is unclear although it is known that GSK3β, which is activated in ACM, can promote inflammation through NFκB signaling.[18-21] Nevertheless, cardiac myocytes in ACM produce and secrete large amounts of diverse chemical mediators of the immune response in a cell-autonomous fashion.[8] Many are powerful chemoattractant molecules that likely mobilize bone marrow-derived inflammatory cells to the heart. Cardiac myocytes in ACM also produce powerful proinflammatory mediators such as IL-1β and TNFα, both of which are considered primordial cytokines of the innate immune response. This suggests that activation of immune signaling within cardiac myocytes may play an important role in driving the key clinical features of the disease. It also raises the interesting possibility that cytokines secreted by cardiac myocytes act in an autocrine fashion to alter ion channel function and promote arrhythmias in ACM. If so, this would add to the traditional view of the role of inflammation in arrhythmogenesis, which holds that cardiac ion channel dysfunction is mediated by cytokines produced by lymphocytes and macrophages that infiltrate the heart in myocarditis or other inflammatory heart diseases.[22]

Our results raise the possibility that targeting immune signaling could be an effective mechanism-based therapy in ACM. This notion is in keeping with recent insights into the role of immune activation in coronary artery disease and heart failure. For example, long-term use of canakinumab, a monoclonal antibody against IL-1β, significantly reduced major adverse cardiac events in patients with coronary artery disease in the CANTOS trail.[23] It also improves outcomes in a dose-dependent fashion in heart failure patients with prior myocardial infarction and elevated high-sensitivity C-reactive protein.[24] The fact that IL-1β expression was increased by ~13-fold in $Dsg2^{mut/mut}$ mice warrants further investigation as a possible therapeutic strategy in ACM. Finally, strenuous exercise is known to accelerate disease penetrance and increase arrhythmic risk in ACM patients.[25,26] It remains to be determined if exercise intensifies the immune response in ACM and, if so, whether anti-inflammatory therapy might mitigate its adverse effects.

Funding Sources

This work was supported by grants from St. Jude Medical (2015–2016 Heart Rhythm Society Cardiac Pacing and Electrophysiology Fellowship Award) and The Aiding Hearts Foundation (to SPC); an American Heart Association Transformational Project Award (18TPA34170559, to SPC and JES); grants from the Gilead Research Scholars in Cardiovascular Disease Fund and the British Heart Foundation (PG/18/27/33616) (to AA); an American Heart Association Pre-doctoral Fellowship Award (to JL); and NIH grant 5R01 HL120959 (to LT). We gratefully acknowledge support for the statistical analysis from the National Center for Research Resources and the National Center for Advancing Translational Sciences (NCATS) of the National Institutes of Health through grant number 1UL1TR001079.

References

1. Marcus FI, Fontaine GH, Guiraudon G, Frank R, Laurenceau JL, Malergue C, Grogogeat Y. Right ventricular dysplasia: A report of 24 adult cases. *Circulation.* 1982;65:384–398.

2. Fontaine G, Fontaliran F, Andrade FR, et al. The arrhythmogenic right ventricle: Dysplasia versus cardiomyopathy. *Heart Vessels.* 1995;10:227–235.

3. Corrado D, Basso C, Thiene G, et al. Spectrum of clinicopathologic manifestations of arrhythmogenic right ventricular cardiomyopathy/dysplasia: A multicenter study. *J Am Coll Cardiol.* 1997;30:1512–1520.

4. Lopez-Ayala JM, Pastor-Quirante F, Gonzalez-Carrillo J, et al. Genetics of myocarditis in arrhythmogenic right ventricular dysplasia. *Heart Rhythm.* 2015;12:766–773.

5. Asimaki A, Tandri H, Duffy ER, et al. Altered desmosomal proteins in granulomatous myocarditis and potential pathogenic links to arrhythmogenic right ventricular cardiomyopathy. *Circ Arrhythm Electrophysiol.* 2011;4:743–752.

6. Campbell JJ, Perkins ND. Regulation of NF-kappaB function. *Biochem Soc Symp.* 2006;73:165–180.

7. Hayden MS, Ghosh S. Shared principles in NF-kappaB signaling. *Cell.* 2008;132:344–362.

8. Chelko SP, Asimaki A, Lowenthal J, et al. Therapeutic modulation of the immune response in arrhythmogenic cardiomyopathy. *Circulation.* 2019;140:1491–1505.

9. Asimaki A, Kapoor S, Plovie E, et al. Identification of a new modulator of the intercalated disc in a zebrafish model of arrhythmogenic cardiomyopathy. *Sci Transl Med.* 2014;240ra74.

10. Chelko SP, Asimaki A, Andersen P, et al. Central role for GSK3β in the pathogenesis of arrhythmogenic cardiomyopathy. *JCI Insight.* 2016;1(5)pii:e85923.

11. Buchman K. Evolution of innate immunity: Clues from invertebrates via fish to mammals. *Front Immunol.* 2014;5:1–8.

12. Gourbal B, Pinaud S, Beckers GJM, Van Der Meer JWM, Conrath U, Netea MG. Innate immune memory: An evolutionary perspective. *Immunol Rev.* 2018;283:21–40.

13. Epelman S, Liu PP, Mann DL. Role of innate and adaptive immunity in cardiac injury and repair. *Nat Rev Immunol.* 2015;15:117–129.

14. Herron BJ, Roa C, Liu S, et al. A mutation in *NFκB interacting protein 1* results in cardiomyopathy and abnormal skin development in *wa3* mice. *Hum Mol Genet.* 2005;14:667–677.

15. Whittington RJ, Cook RW. Cardiomyopathy and woolly haircoat syndrome of Poll Hereford cattle: Electrocardiographic findings in affected and unaffected calves. *Austral Vet J.* 1988;65:341–344.

16. Simpson MA, Cook RW, Solanki P, Patton MA, Dennis JA, Crosby AH. A mutation in *NFκB interacting protein 1* causes cardiomyopathy and woolly haircoat in Poll Hereford cattle. *Animal Genet.* 2008;40:42–46.

17. Basso C, Thiene G, Corrado D, Angelini A, Nava A, Valente M. Arrhythmogenic right ventricular cardiomyopathy: Dysplasia, dystrophy or myocarditis? *Circulation.* 1996;94:983–991.

18. Takada Y, Fang X, Jamaluddin MS, Boyd DD, Aggarwal BB. Genetic deletion of glycogen synthase kinase-3beta abrogates activation of IkappaBalpha kinase, JNK, Akt, and p44/p42 MAPK but potentiates apoptosis induced by tumor necrosis factor. *J Biol Chem.* 2004;279:39541–39554.

19. Fiol CJ, Williams JS, Chou CH, Wang QM, Roach PJ, Andrisani OM. A secondary phosphorylation of CREB341 at Ser129 is required for the cAMP-mediated control of gene expression: A role for glycogen synthase kinase-3 in the control of gene expression. *J Biol Chem.* 1994;269:32187–32193.

20. Bullock BP, Habener JF. Phosphorylation of the cAMP response element binding protein CREB by cAMP dependent protein kinase A and glycogen synthase kinase-3 alters DNA binding affinity, conformation, and increases net charge. *Biochemistry.* 1998;37:3795–3809.

21. Martin M, Rehani K, Jope RS, Michalek SM. Toll-like receptor-mediated cytokine production is differentially regulated by glycogen synthase kinase 3. *Nat Immunol.* 2005;6:777–784.

22. Lazzerini PE, Capecchi PL, Laghi-Pasini F. Systemic inflammation and arrhythmic risk: Lessons from rheumatoid arthritis. *Eur Heart J.* 2017;38:1717–1727.

23. Ridker PR, Everett BM, Thuren T, et al. Anti-inflammatory therapy with canakinumab for atherosclerotic disease. *N Eng J Med.* 2017;377:1119–1131.

24. Everett BM, Cornel JH, Lainscak M, et al. Anti-inflammatory therapy with canakinumab for the prevention of hospitalization for heart failure. *Circulation.* 2019;139:1289–1299.

25. James, CA, Bhonsale A, Tichnell C, et al. Exercise increases age-related penetrance and arrhythmic risk in arrhythmogenic right ventricular dysplasia/cardiomyopathy-associated desmosomal mutation carriers. *J Am Coll Cardiol.* 2013;62:1290–1297.

26. Rojas A, Calkins H. Present understanding of the relationship between exercise and arrhythmogenic right ventricular dysplasia/cardiomyopathy. *Trends Cardiovasc Med.* 2015;25:181–188.

5

Studying Arrhythmogenic Cardiomyopathy Under the Microscope

Monica De Gaspari, MD; Stefania Rizzo, MD, PhD; Gaetano Thiene, MD; Cristina Basso, MD, PhD

Introduction

Arrhythmogenic right ventricular cardiomyopathy (ARVC) is an inherited heart muscle disease characterized by fibrofatty replacement of the myocardium at risk of life-threatening electrical instability.[1–5] It was initially considered a developmental defect of the right ventricular (RV) myocardium, that is, a congenital malformation, as recalled by the original name "RV dysplasia."[6] Only in the late 1980s was the heredo-familial background, with an autosomal dominant transmission and variable penetrance,[7] recognized, and the disease was eventually listed among cardiomyopathies in 1995.[4] In the new millennium, the genetic background[5] has been clarified, with up to 50% of probands affected carrying one or more mutations in genes encoding for desmosomal proteins. More recently, by performing cardiac magnetic resonance (CMR) imaging in genotyped patients and detailed pathology examination, it has also been demonstrated that the disease is not anymore exclusive to the RV, thus leading to the denomination of arrhythmogenic cardiomyopathy (AC) to include the biventricular and left-dominant variants besides the traditional ARVC.[8–13]

Pathological Anatomy of ARVC

The first systematic description of morphological abnormalities of ARVC dates back to 1988, when full hearts coming from the autopsies of young persons who suffered sudden cardiac death (SCD) in northeastern Italy were investigated.[2] At that time, the disease was recognized as another cause, besides hypertrophic cardiomyopathy (HCM), of cardiac arrest in the young and in athletes. According to the original definition, the pathologic diagnosis of ARVC was based upon gross and histologic evidence of transmural myocardial atrophy in the RV free wall, extending from the epicardium towards the endocardium.[4] RV aneurysms located in the so-called triangle of dysplasia (i.e., inflow, apex, and outflow tract) were considered a pathognomonic feature of ARVC (**Figure 5.1**).[2,3] A higher prevalence of biventricular involvement, usually with ventricular chamber dilatation, multiple aneurysms, and a parchment-like appearance of the thinned free wall, was reported in cases with end-stage disease and congestive heart failure as clinical presentation.[3,14]

Histological examination revealed islands of surviving myocytes interspersed with fibrous and fatty tissue.[2,3,14] At that time, a lipomatous variant was also recognized. However, it has been thereafter demonstrated that RV fatty infiltration is not a sufficient morphologic hallmark of ARVC,[15] since a certain amount of intramyocardial fat is physiologically present in the RV free wall, particularly in the antero-lateral and apical regions, and increases with age and body size. Furthermore, ARVC should not be confused

with adipositas cordis due to increased epicardial fat typically observed in obese people.[15] Replacement-type fibrosis and cardiomyocyte (CM) degenerative changes are thus essential to provide a clearcut diagnosis of ARVC, besides fatty tissue replacement.

Since the beginning, it was appreciated that these histopathological features shared similarities with those observed in skeletal muscle dystrophies (such as Duchenne's or Becker's), that is, a progressive and acquired muscular atrophy with replacement by exuberant fatty and fibrous tissue.[3] Thus, in ARVC, CM death, either by apoptosis or by necrosis, could account for a genetically determined progressive loss of the ventricular myocardium.[3,16,17] The discovery of the first disease gene (plakoglobin) opened the door to the identification of additional genes in the autosomal dominant variants of ARVC, that is, desmoplakin, plakophilin-2, desmoglein-2, and desmocollin-2.[5]

Inflammatory cells, probably reactive in nature, were reported in up to two-thirds of

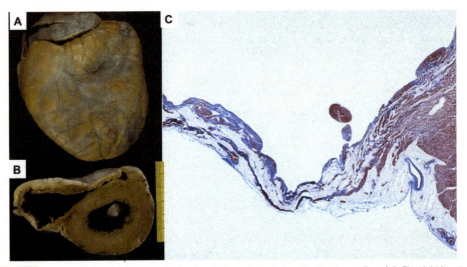

FIGURE 5.1   Diffuse ARVC in a 14-year-old athlete who died suddenly during effort is shown. **Panel A:** The right heart appears dilated and yellow with anterior aneurysm. **Panel B:** Anterior and posterior RV aneurysms and focal left ventricular (LV) free wall involvement are appreciable on cross section. **Panel C:** Transmural fibrofatty replacement at the level of RV aneurysm is shown.

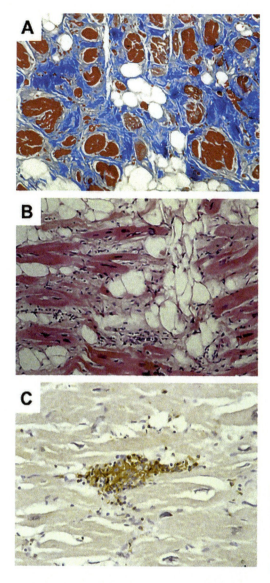

FIGURE 5.2 Histological features of ARVC include the following: surviving myocytes entrapped within fibrous and fatty tissue (**Panel A**); adipocytes, fibroblasts, and inflammatory infiltrates (**Panel B**); and positive T-lymphocytes at immunohistochemistry (**Panel C**).

cases at histology,[18] raising the issue of myocarditis role in disease pathogenesis (**Figure 5.2**).

Notably, in the late 1990s there was still a lot of confusion about the pathomorphology of ARVC, in part created by the misuse of the term *Uhl's anomaly*, originally reported as "an almost total absence of the myocardium of the RV" in a 7-month-old infant.[19] However, while in Uhl's anomaly the epicardium was directly in contact with the endocardium in the absence of myocardium and intervening fat, in ARVC there was always fibrofatty tissue with interspersed residual CMs between the epicardial and endocardial layers. Differential diagnosis criteria included the lack of family history, the clinical presentation with heart failure rather than arrhythmias, and the age of presentation, usually in childhood for Uhl's anomaly.

From ARVC to AC, Recognizing the Wider Phenotypic Spectrum

All of the above mentioned morphologic features refer to the classical ARVC variant. With the advent of CMR and extensive histopathological studies of hearts coming from either autopsy or heart transplantation (HTx), it has been demonstrated that the disease can show a spectrum of morphological abnormalities much wider than previously thought. Moreover, the source of cases can also influence the results, since some published series are mostly based on cases coming from referral centers for arrhythmias/sudden death and others for heart failure/cardiac transplantation.

Thus, besides ARVC with aneurysms in the triangle of dysplasia, grossly normal hearts in whom only a careful histopathology investigation can reveal the myocardial changes, not necessarily transmural (**Figure 5.3**), and hearts with isolated or dominant LV involvement (**Figure 5.4**) have been reported and described under the common umbrella of ACM.[1,10]

Obviously, histopathologic features mostly depend on the entry selection criteria. Since "transmural fibrofatty myocardial replacement of the RV free wall" has been considered a requirement for the pathologic diagnosis of ARVC,[4] many cases with early and focal RV involvement or those with dominant or isolated LV disease, without aneurysm formation, escaped the diagnosis.

Recently, Chen et al. constructed a novel pathological classification of AC through unsupervised algorithm based on circumferential fibrofatty tissue distribution, beyond the traditional distinction into *isolated RV, biventricular, and LV dominant subtypes*. The most striking discovery was that this novel classification possesses distinctive genetic backgrounds, suggesting that genotype plays an essential role in determining pathological expression.[20]

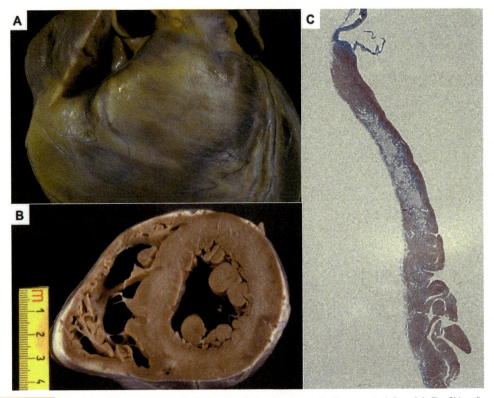

FIGURE 5.3 Segmental ARVC in a 26-year-old athlete who died suddenly on effort is presented. **Panel A:** The RV outflow tract is mildly dilated. **Panel B:** No aneurysms are visible on cross section but only a focal involvement of the posterior RV free wall. **Panel C:** Histology of the RV outflow tract shows the regional fibrofatty replacement.

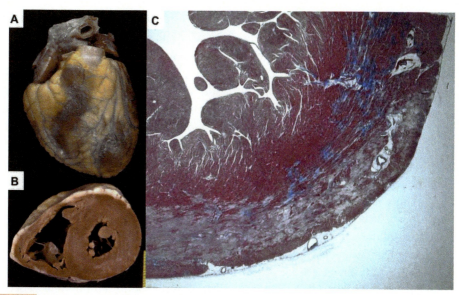

FIGURE 5.4 Early AC with myocarditis-like presentation in a 14-year-old boy who died suddenly at rest (family member, *DSP* mutation carrier). **Panel A:** Normal appearance of the heart at external examination. **Panel B:** No aneurysms are visible on cross section but only a focal involvement of the posterior RV free wall. **Panel C:** Subepicardial injury with inflammation and necrosis at histology of the LV free wall is shown.

Observations in human patients as well as in experimental animal models suggest that the disease progression, rather than being a continuous process, may occur during periodic "bursts" of an otherwise stable disease, which can be clinically silent but sometimes may be characterized by life-threatening arrhythmic exacerbation.[8,21–23] These bursts leading to disease onset and progression may be either spontaneous or triggered by environmental factors, such as exercise or inflammation.

Since the original descriptions, it has been a matter of debate whether the inflammatory cells are reactive to cell death or the consequence of infective or immune mechanisms.[3,16] Although cardiotropic viruses have been reported in the myocardium of some ARVC patients, and they have been proposed as possible etiologic agents to support an infective pathogenesis,[24,25] the viruses might be just innocent bystanders or play a secondary important role. In other words, the atrophic myocardium could favor the viral settlement

with superimposed myocarditis, leading to disease progression. Notably, inflammatory cell infiltrates have been described both in spontaneous animal models and in transgenic animal models, which supports the reactive nature of myocarditis.[22,26]

With the recognition of the genetic background leading to the concept of ARVC as a disease of the desmosome, morphologic and molecular studies of intercellular junctions became a major issue both in humans and in experimental pathology.[27–30]

Ultrastructural investigation of endomyocardial biopsies (EMB) in gene-positive ARVC patients revealed intercalated disk remodeling,[29] so that the number of desmosomes was significantly lower, the desmosomal gap widened, and the desmosomal length was higher in ARVC than in controls. Abnormally located desmosomes with pale internal plaques were also identified in most of the cases; immunohistochemical and molecular studies demonstrated plakoglobin redistribution from the intercellular junctions in Naxos disease and Carvajal syndrome,[27,28] providing the first evidence that a desmosomal gene mutation may perturb the subcellular distribution of other intercellular junction proteins although not genetically altered. Asimaki et al.[30] found that the plakoglobin signal was diminished at intercalated disks and appeared to be relatively specific for ARVC, thus suggesting that the immunohistochemical evaluation of desmosomal proteins on EMB could represent a promising diagnostic test for ARVC. Redistribution of plakoglobin from junctions to intracellular pools could be part of a final common pathway in disease pathogenesis, and impaired mechanical coupling might account for abnormal electrical coupling by gap junction remodeling. However, the test did not enter the routine diagnostic workup due to false negative and positive results and absence of reproducibility across various pathology labs.

Nonischemic LV Scar

Arrhythmogenic LV Cardiomyopathy vs. Myocarditis

The increasing use of contrast-enhanced CMR in genotyped patients, together with more extensive pathology examination of heart specimens of people dying suddenly, led to the recognition in the last decade of subepicardial and/or midmural fibrosis, in the absence of (or unrelated to) significant coronary artery disease (the so-called nonischemic left ventricular scar [NLVS]; **Figure 5.5**). Genotype-phenotype correlation allowed us to conclude that this entity can be part of the phenotypic spectrum of AC, although some can be the sequela of previous myocarditis.[8,12,31–33]

In a series of consecutive cases of juvenile sudden death, NLVS was the most frequent finding (25%) in those occurring during sports.[30] The scar was localized most frequently within the LV posterior wall and affected the subepicardial myocardium, often extending to the midventricular layer. On histology, it consisted of fibrous or fibrofatty tissue, RV involvement was always present, and patchy lymphocytic infiltrates were frequent. Autopsy study and clinical screening of family members are required to differentiate between AC and chronic acquired myocarditis.

Furthermore, in a recent series of 202 cases diagnosed with AC at postmortem, LV histopathologic involvement was found in 87% of cases and was isolated in 17%.[33] The most common areas of fibrofatty infiltration were the LV posterobasal (68%) and anterolateral walls (58%). Postmortem genetic testing yielded pathogenic variants in AC-related genes in 25% of decedents.

Role of Transvenous Endomyocardial Biopsy

EMB may be of great help in the diagnostic workup for an *in vivo tissue characterization through* histological demonstration of fibrofatty myocardial replacement.[34–37] In fact, the 2010 International Task Force Criteria (TFC) still recognize the role of this diagnostic tool.[37] Samples should be retrieved from the free wall, since the RV fibrofatty replacement is usually transmural and thus detectable from the endocardium, whereas the septum is often spared by the disease. A residual amount of myocardium < 60%, due to fibrous or fibrofatty replacement, has a high diagnostic accuracy and is now listed among major diagnostic criteria for ARVC. To improve the diagnostic sensitivity, an EMB procedure guided either by electro-anatomic mapping or by CMR has been suggested.[38] EMB is essential to rule out the so-called AC "phenocopies," such as myocarditis, sarcoidosis, or idiopathic RV outflow tract tachycardia, particularly when dealing with probands with a sporadic ARVC form.[39-42]

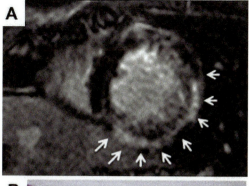

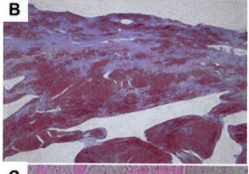

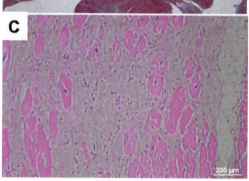

FIGURE 5.5 The heart of an 18-year-old athlete with NLVS who developed heart failure at follow-up is shown.
Panel A: CMR reveals subepicardial/midmyocardial late gadolinium enhancement with a stria pattern involving the inferolateral LV wall (**white arrows**).
Panel B: Panoramic view of the inferolateral LV free wall of the explanted heart at transplantation is presented; extensive replacement-type fibrosis appears mostly in the subepicardial and midmural layers, with focal fatty infiltration.
Panel C: At higher magnification, CMs with dysmetric and dysmorphic nuclei, cytoplasmic vacuolization, and diffuse fibrosis with patchy fatty infiltration are shown.

The increasing recognition of left-dominant or even isolated LV variants raises the issue of the diagnostic role of EMB and of the need to introduce contrast-enhanced CMR for tissue characterization among diagnostic criteria in the category of tissue characterization.[43] The subepicardial/midmural involvement and the RV approach explain the frequent negative findings in this setting. Notably, in the series of athletes with NLVS and life-threatening arrhythmias, EMB provided normal histologic findings in 50% of cases, while in the remainder it was consistent with focal acute myocarditis or segmental fibrofatty replacement. Molecular pathology investigation by polymerase chain reaction and reverse-transcriptase polymerase chain reaction was negative for viral genomes.[32]

References

1. Basso C, Corrado D, Marcus FI, Nava A, Thiene G. Arrhythmogenic right ventricular cardiomyopathy. *Lancet.* 2009;373:1289–1300.

2. Thiene G, Nava A, Corrado D, Rossi L, Pennelli N. Right ventricular cardiomyopathy and sudden death in young people. *N Engl J Med.* 1988;318:129–133.

3. Basso C, Thiene G, Corrado D, Angelini A, Nava A, Valente M. Arrhythmogenic

right ventricular cardiomyopathy: Dysplasia, dystrophy or myocarditis? *Circulation.* 1996;94:983–991.

4. Richardson P, McKenna W, Bristow M, et al. Report of the 1995 World Health Organization/International Society and Federation of Cardiology Task Force on the definition and classification of cardiomyopathies. *Circulation.* 1996;93:841–842.

5. Pilichou K, Thiene G, Bauce B, et al. Arrhythmogenic cardiomyopathy. *Orphanet J Rare Dis.* 2016;11:33.

6. Basso C, Corrado D, Thiene G. Arrhythmogenic right ventricular cardiomyopathy: What's in a name? From a congenital defect (dysplasia) to a genetically determined cardiomyopathy (dystrophy). *Am J Cardiol.* 2010;106:275–277.

7. Nava A, Thiene G, Canciani B, et al. Familial occurrence of right ventricular dysplasia: A study involving nine families. *J Am Coll Cardiol.* 1989;12:1222–1228.

8. Bauce B, Basso C, Rampazzo A, et al. Clinical profile of four families with arrhythmogenic right ventricular cardiomyopathy caused by dominant desmoplakin mutations. *Eur Heart J.* 2005;26:1666–1675.

9. Sen-Chowdhry S, Syrris P, Prasad SK, et al. Left-dominant arrhythmogenic cardiomyopathy: An under-recognized clinical entity. *J Am Coll Cardiol.* 2008;52:2175–2187.

10. Basso C, Bauce B, Corrado D, Thiene G. Pathophysiology of arrhythmogenic cardiomyopathy. *Nat Rev Cardiol.* 2011;9:223–233.

11. Marra MP, Leoni L, Bauce B, et al. Imaging study of ventricular scar in arrhythmogenic right ventricular cardiomyopathy: Comparison of 3D standard electroanatomical voltage mapping and contrast-enhanced cardiac magnetic resonance. *Circ Arrhythm Electrophysiol.* 2012;5(1):91–100.

12. Pilichou K, Mancini M, Rigato I, et al. Nonischemic left ventricular scar: Sporadic or familial? Screen the genes, scan the mutation carriers. *Circulation.* 2014;130:e180–e182.

13. Cipriani A, Bauce B, De Lazzari M, et al. Arrhythmogenic right ventricular cardiomyopathy: Characterization of left ventricular phenotype and differential diagnosis with dilated cardiomyopathy. *J Am Heart Assoc.* 2020 Mar 3;9(5):e014628.

14. Corrado D, Basso C, Thiene G, et al. Spectrum of clinicopathologic manifestations of arrhythmogenic right ventricular cardiomyopathy/dysplasia: a multicenter study. *J Am Coll Cardiol.* 1997; 30:1512–1520.

15. Basso C, Thiene G. Adipositas cordis, fatty infiltration of the right ventricle, and arrhythmogenic right ventricular cardiomyopathy. Just a matter of fat? *Cardiovasc Pathol.* 2005;14:37–41.

16. Mallat Z, Tedgui A, Fontaliran F, Frank R, Durigon M, Fontaine G. Evidence of apoptosis in arrhythmogenic right ventricular dysplasia. *N Engl J Med.* 1996;335:1190–1196.

17. Valente M, Calabrese F, Thiene G, Angelini A, Basso C, Nava A, Rossi L. In vivo evidence of apoptosis in arrhythmogenic right ventricular cardiomyopathy. *Am J Pathol.* 1998;152:479–484.

18. Thiene G, Corrado D, Nava A, et al. Right ventricular cardiomyopathy: Is there evidence of an inflammatory aetiology? *Eur Heart J.* 1991;12:22–25.

19. Uhl HS. A previously undescribed congenital malformation of the heart: Almost total absence of the myocardium of the right ventricle. *Bull Johns Hopkins Hosp.* 1952;91:197–209.

20. Chen L, Song J, Chen X, et al. A novel genotype-based clinicopathology classification of arrhythmogenic cardiomyopathy provides novel insights into disease progression. *Eur Heart J.* 2019;40(21):1690–1703.

21. Nava A, Bauce B, Basso C, et al. Clinical profile and long-term follow-up of 37 families with arrhythmogenic right ventricular cardiomyopathy. *J Am Coll Cardiol.* 2000;36:2226–2233.

22. Pilichou K, Remme CA, Basso C, et al. Myocyte necrosis underlies progressive myocardial dystrophy in mouse dsg2-related arrhythmogenic right ventricular cardiomyopathy. *J Exp Med.* 2009;206:1787–1802.

23. Zorzi A, Rigato I, Pilichou K, et al. Phenotypic expression is a prerequisite for malignant

arrhythmic events and sudden cardiac death in arrhythmogenic right ventricular cardiomyopathy. *Europace*. 2016;18:1086–1094.

24. Bowles NE, Ni J, Marcus F, Towbin JA. The detection of cardiotropic viruses in the myocardium of patients with arrhythmogenic right ventricular dysplasia/cardiomyopathy. *J Am Coll Cardiol*. 2002;39:892–895.

25. Calabrese F, Basso C, Carturan E, Valente M, Thiene G. Arrhythmogenic right ventricular cardiomyopathy/dysplasia: Is there a role for viruses? *Cardiovasc Pathol*. 2006;15:11–17.

26. Fox PR, Maron BJ, Basso C, Liu SK, Thiene G: Spontaneously occurring arrhythmogenic right ventricular cardiomyopathy in the domestic cat: A new animal model similar to the human disease. *Circulation*. 2000;102:1863–1870.

27. Kaplan SR, Gard JJ, Protonotarios N, et al. Remodeling of myocyte gap junctions in arrhythmogenic right ventricular cardiomyopathy due to a deletion in plakoglobin (Naxos disease). *Heart Rhythm*. 2004;1:3–11.

28. Kaplan SR, Gard JJ, Carvajal-Huerta L, Ruiz-Cabezas JC, Thiene G, Saffitz JE. Structural and molecular pathology of the heart in Carvajal syndrome. *Cardiovasc Pathol*. 2004;13:26–32.

29. Basso C, Czarnowska E, Della Barbera M, et al. Ultrastructural evidence of intercalated disc remodelling in arrhythmogenic right ventricular cardiomyopathy: An electron microscopy investigation on endomyocardial biopsies. *Eur Heart J*. 2006;27:1847–1854.

30. Asimaki A, Tandri H, Huang H, et al. A new diagnostic test for arrhythmogenic right ventricular cardiomyopathy. *N Engl J Med*. 2009;360:1075–1084.

31. di Gioia CR, Giordano C, Cerbelli B, et al. Nonischemic left ventricular scar and cardiac sudden death in the young. *Hum Pathol*. 2016;58:78–89.

32. Zorzi A, Perazzolo Marra M, Rigato I, et al. Nonischemic left ventricular scar as a substrate of life-threatening ventricular arrhythmias and sudden cardiac death in competitive athletes. *Circ Arrhythm Electrophysiol*. 2016;9:e004229.

33. Miles C, Finocchiaro G, Papadakis M, et al. Sudden death and left ventricular involvement in arrhythmogenic cardiomyopathy. *Circulation*. 2019;139(15):1786–1797.

34. McKenna WJ, Thiene G, Nava A, et al. Diagnosis of arrhythmogenic right ventricular dysplasia/cardiomyopathy. Task Force of the Working Group Myocardial and Pericardial Disease of the European Society of Cardiology and of the Scientific Council on Cardiomyopathies of the International Society and Federation of Cardiology. *Br Heart J*. 1994;71:215–218.

35. Angelini A, Basso C, Nava A, Thiene G. Endomyocardial biopsy in arrhythmogenic right ventricular cardiomyopathy. *Am Heart J*. 1996;132:203–206.

36. Basso C, Ronco F, Marcus F, et al. Quantitative assessment of endomyocardial biopsy in arrhythmogenic right ventricular cardiomyopathy/dysplasia: An in vitro validation of diagnostic criteria. *Eur Heart J*. 2008;29:2760–2771.

37. Marcus FI, McKenna WJ, Sherrill D, et al. Diagnosis of arrhythmogenic right ventricular cardiomyopathy/dysplasia: Proposed modification of the Task Force Criteria. *Circulation*. 2010;121:1533–1541.

38. Casella M, Dello Russo A, Bergonti M, et al. Diagnostic yield of electroanatomic voltage mapping in guiding endomyocardial biopsies. *Circulation*. 2020;142(13):1249–1260.

39. Corrado D, Basso C, Leoni L, et al. Three-dimensional electroanatomical voltage mapping and histologic evaluation of myocardial substrate in right ventricular outflow tract tachycardia. *J Am Coll Cardiol*. 2008;51:731–739.

40. Corrado D, Basso C, Leoni L, et al. Three-dimensional electroanatomic voltage mapping increases accuracy of diagnosing arrhythmogenic right ventricular cardiomyopathy/dysplasia. *Circulation*. 2005;111:3042–3050.

41. Ladyjanskaia GA, Basso C, Hobbelink MG, et al. Sarcoid myocarditis with ventricular tachycardia mimicking ARVD/C. *J Cardiovasc Electrophysiol*. 2010;21:94–98.

42. Vasaiwala SC, Finn C, Delpriore J, et al. Prospective study of cardiac sarcoid mimicking arrhythmogenic right ventricular dysplasia. *J Cardiovasc Electrophysiol.* 2009;20:473–476.

43. Corrado D, Perazzolo Marra M, Zorzi A, et al. Diagnosis of arrhythmogenic cardiomyopathy: The Padua criteria. *Int J Cardiol.* 2020:S0167-5273(20)33293-9.

6

Genetic Contributions to Arrhythmogenic Cardiomyopathy

Daniel P. Judge, MD; J. Peter van Tintelen, MD, PhD

Introduction

Arrhythmogenic cardiomyopathy (ACM) is widely recognized as an inherited form of heart disease. From the earliest descriptions of this uncommon form of cardiomyopathy with fibrofatty scar, the pattern of familial occurrence indicated a Mendelian disorder.[1,2] The earliest approach for gene identification relied on traditional chromosomal linkage analysis in families with multiple affected individuals followed by direct sequencing of potential interesting genes. This was the most common technique used until approximately 15 years ago. Unfortunately, small families and frequent lack of affected individuals due to early sudden cardiac death (SCD) led to few pedigrees large enough to have informative linkage analysis. Low penetrance also impaired proper assignment of chromosomal loci harboring the responsible genes. However, more efficient DNA sequencing technology with

lower costs later led to many important discoveries. Recognition of the earliest genes involved with ACM naturally identified other candidate genes encoding related proteins. This chapter will focus on the initial research that characterized syndromic forms of ACM, subsequent desmosomal and nondesmosomal genes involved with ACM, the relevance of genetic testing in routine clinical practice, and the likely direction of future research that tries to identify the genetic basis of ACM.

Syndromic ACM

Dr. Nikos Protonotarios and his wife, Dr. Adalena Tsatsopoulou, first reported a recessive disorder that they named Naxos disease due to its occurrence on that Greek island.[3] Affected individuals had palmoplantar keratoderma, woolly hair, and cardiac enlargement with anterior precordial T-wave inversion on electrocardiograms (ECGs), and most had syncope or ventricular tachycardia (VT). Naxos disease was unique among the familial nonepi-dermolytic palmoplantar keratodermas known at the time, in that those with Naxos disease also had cardiac problems, which co-segregated with the skin and hair abnormalities. Pedigree analysis fit best with an autosomal recessive disorder, and genome-wide linkage analysis with homozygosity mapping identified a 7-centimorgan region on chromosome 17q21.[4] Fine-resolution mapping narrowed the interval to 0.7 centimorgans, containing *JUP*, encoding the desmosome protein junction plakoglobin.[5] Further analysis of this candidate gene identified deletion of 2 nucleotides, resulting in a frameshift and premature termination of the plakoglobin protein. All affected individuals were homozygous for this deletion, and heterozygous family members were phenotypically unaffected.[5] This important initial observation set the stage for analysis of many related genes encoding other elements in the cardiac desmosome.

A few years later, a dermatologist in Ecuador, Dr. Luis Carvajal-Huerta, reported a similar syndrome.[6] Over nearly 3 decades, he found 18 people with palmoplantar keratoderma, woolly hair, and dilated cardiomyopathy. Pedigree analysis indicated a recessive genetic disorder, and homozygosity mapping identified a recessive frameshift mutation in *DSP*, encoding desmoplakin, another protein of the cardiac desmosome.[7] Because desmoplakin and plakoglobin are both components of the cardiac desmosome, their associations with Carvajal syndrome and Naxos disease (respectively) set the stage for candidate gene analysis, focusing on other components of the cardiac desmosome.

Nonsyndromic Desmosomal ACM

Several chromosomal loci have been associated with arrhythmogenic right ventricular cardiomyopathy (ARVC), the right-dominant subtype of ACM, in attempts to identify other genetic contributions to this disorder.[8-14] Unfortunately, those studies were complicated by a relatively high percentage of affected individuals in large families having early SCD, without available DNA. Also, low penetrance and uncertainty in phenotypic assignment for family members with nonspecific abnormalities led to errors or absence of a gene with pathogenic variants linked to ARVC within the assigned genomic intervals (**Table 6.1**). Starting with ARVD8, as designated in the Online Mendelian Inheritance in Man (OMIM) database, candidate gene sequencing was the primary modality used for assignment of additional chromosomal loci.

After publication of the causes for Naxos disease and Carvajal syndrome, investigators in Italy reported a heterozygous mutation in *DSP* in a single family, which altered binding between desmoplakin and plakoglobin, resulting in a dominant form of nonsyndromic ARVC.[15] These investigators later identified additional families segregating other dominant *DSP* mutations with ARVC, noting that left ventricular (LV) involvement often also occurs in these families.[16] The next major discovery in unraveling the genetic basis for ACM involved a large multicenter analysis of 120 unrelated probands with this condition.[17] The investigators chose *PKP2* as a candidate gene, because its encoded protein (plakophilin-2) is a member of the cardiac desmosome, and because of embryonic lethality with cardiac defects in *Pkp2*-null mice.[18] Remarkably, 32 of 120 (27%) had heterozygous variants in *PKP2* that were deemed pathogenic.[17] Among these, 4 were missense variants, and 28 were truncating or frame-shift variants. At least one of the missense variants (*PKP2* p.Ser140Phe, rs150821281) was later reported as relatively common (MAF 0.002), and not associated with heart failure, arrhythmia, premature death, or ARVC.[19]

TABLE 6.1   Chromosomal Loci for ARVC

NAME	OMIM#	CHROMOSOME	GENE
ARVD1	107970	14q24.3	*TGFB3*
ARVD2	600996	1q43	*RYR2*
ARVD3	602086	14q12–q22	
ARVD4	602087	2q32.1–q32.3	
ARVD5	604400	3p25	*TMEM43*
ARVD6	604401	10p12–p14	
ARVD7	609160	10q22.3	revised to chr.2q35 and *DES*
ARVD8	607450	6p24.3	*DSP*
ARVD9	609040	12p11.21	*PKP2*
ARVD10	610193	18q12.1	*DSG2*
ARVD11	610476	18q12.1	*DSC2*
ARVD12	611528	17q21.1	*JUP*
ARVD13	615616	10q21.3	*CTNNA3*

The prevalence of pathogenic variants in *PKP2* among people with ARVC ranges in different reports from 11%–43%, probably due to differences in phenotypic assignment among expert centers and the presence of mutations originating from an ancient founder in specific populations.[20–22] Focusing on probands with additional affected family members, one study identified that 70% carried a pathogenic *PKP2* variant.[20] Another showed that the presence of a pathogenic *PKP2* variant in people with ARVC correlates with earlier onset of symptoms and arrhythmia.[21] There are 4 different plakophilins, although p0071 (*PKP4*) localizes to the adherens junctions rather than desmosomes.[23] The other 2 plakophilins, *PKP1* and *PKP3*, are not well expressed in myocardium, where plakophilin-2 serves as the predominant cardiac subtype.[24] Redundancy by other plakophilins in the skin may explain the paucity of dermal manifestations in people with heterozygous abnormalities in *PKP2*.

Investigation of other candidate genes related to the cardiac desmosome led to recognition of *DSG2* as a gene harboring mutations that predispose to ARVC. Two groups simulta-neously reported 12 unrelated probands with 1 or 2 pathogenic variants in this gene encoding desmoglein-2, accounting for 12%–15% of those without mutations in *DSP* or *PKP2*.[25,26] As with the plakophilins, there are 4 different members of the desmoglein family, with *DSG2* expressed as the predominant type in the heart, while the others play a more important part in skin.[27] Using a similar candidate-gene approach, 2 separate groups reported that *DSC2* mutations cause ARVC.[28,29] These reports included a cumulative 165 probands without a discernible genetic cause for their ARVC, finding 3 (1.8%) with pathogenic variants in *DSC2*. Finally, the desmosomal gene linked to recessive Naxos disease, *JUP*, was subsequently demonstrated to have heterozygous mutations that cause nonsyndromic, autosomal dominantly inherited ARVC, although this is the least commonly associated cardiac desmosome gene for people with ARVC.[30]

Groups in Europe and North America published most of the early desmosome data in ACM and ARVC in particular, and most of the North American cohorts had a majority of Caucasians with European ancestry. Analysis of 3 large ARVC registries in America and Europe identified that *de novo* variants in the 5 main cardiac desmosome genes are exceedingly uncommon (< 1%), and this investigation did not include paternity testing.[31] Haplotype analysis supports remote common founders for many of the more common pathogenic desmosome variants.[31] Because more than half of the world's population lives in Asia, complementary testing there is helping to augment knowledge of this condition. Studies in China have shown a similar distribution of desmosome gene mutations in people with ACM, although there are differences. For instance, among 118 unrelated Chinese probands with ACM, approximately 40% had pathogenic desmosome variants, consisting of 18.6% in *PKP2*, 15.3% in *DSG2*, 4.2% in *DSP*, and 1.7% in *DSC2*.[32] Approximately 10% in this cohort had the same homozygous pathogenic *DSG2* variant, p.Phe531Cys.[32]

Nondesmosomal ACM

The area composita is a complex of junctional proteins, which includes both the desmosome and the adherens junction.[33] Because of its close proximity and similar function to the desmosome, abnormalities in genes encoding elements of the area composita became robust candidates for contributors to ARVC. In a cohort of 76 Italian probands with ARVC and without pathogenic variants in *PKP2*, *DSP*, *DSG2*, *DSC2*, or *JUP*, one group analyzed *CTNNA3*, encoding alpha-T-catenin.[34] They identified 2 separate probands with rare variants, which are predicted to disrupt cell adhesion.

In a separate line of investigation, a large family in Newfoundland was initially reported in 1988 with an autosomal dominant pattern of inheritance of ARVC.[35] Traditional linkage analysis localized this disorder to the short arm of chromosome 3 at 3p25, and narrowing of the genomic interval occurred due to partici-

pation of many affected individuals spanning several generations.[36,37] Analysis of 20 genes in the linked interval, with additional refinement based on co-segregation analysis, eventually identified a missense variant in *TMEM43*, p.Ser358Leu.[38] Extending beyond Newfoundland, Canada, an international collaboration involving sites in both North America and Europe found a common haplotype, that helps to pinpoint this mutation as occurring between 52 and 64 generations ago.[39] Assuming 25 years per generation, this particular haplotype probably arose in the years 400–700 AD. Recently, additional families have been identified with this identical mutation.[40]

TMEM43 encodes Luma, a nuclear envelope protein, which is part of the LINC (linker of nucleoskeleton and cytoskeleton) complex.[41] Luma binds to both emerin and lamin A/C, and pathogenic variants in both *EMD* and *LMNA* cause a similar constellation of ACM with or without skeletal myopathy.[41] Although *EMD* mutations rarely explain ACM without skeletal muscle disease, the prevalence of pathogenic variants in *LMNA* among people with ACM varies based on the specific phenotype under investigation. For instance, among people with nonischemic dilated cardiomyopathy (DCM), conduction disease, and elevation of serum creatine kinase, *LMNA* mutations are commonly identified, whereas they occur less commonly among people with isolated ARVC.[42,43]

Extending from the concept that abnormalities in the nuclear envelope can cause ACM, homozygous mutations in *LEMD2* also cause ACM.[44,45] This discovery began with investigation of Hutterite trios with recessive cataracts. The Hutterite community originated in Europe in the 16th century and emigrated to North America in the 1870s.[44] Their communities remain mostly genetically isolated. Whole exome sequencing with autozygosity mapping localized the disease locus to a 9.5-Mb region of chromosome 6p21, and additional analysis refined the locus to *LEMD2*.[45] Phenotypic characterization identified high rates of sudden cardiac arrest, and ACM with mild ventricular dysfunction but high rates of ventricular tachyarrhythmias.[44] *LEMD2* encodes a LEM-domain protein, which binds to nuclear lamin A/C and influences proliferation and senescence of cardiac fibroblasts.[44]

One of the early linkage studies identified *RyR2* mutations as responsible for ARVD2.[9,46] The cardiac ryanodine receptor is important for regulation of calcium flux in cardiomyocytes (CMs), and loss of function mutations cause catecholaminergic polymorphic ventricular tachycardia (CPVT).[47] However, most people with CPVT do not have cardiomyopathy, unless it occurs secondarily after cardiac arrest or due to frequent sustained tachyarrhythmias. Although individuals with CPVT may have met early Task Force Criteria (TFC) for ARVC, the absence of structural heart involvement leads most experts not to consider *RyR2* mutations as part of the genetic contributions to ACM. Pathogenic variants in another calcium-regulating protein, phospholamban, do cause structural cardiomyopathy, affecting the right, left, or both ventricles. Studies of ACM in Greece identified three different pathogenic variants in *PLN*, which cause DCM and prominent ventricular arrhythmias (VAs), best characterized as ACM.[48-50] In Holland, a prominent *PLN* founder mutation, p.Arg14del, is present in 10%–15% of people with ACM.[51]

For individuals in whom skeletal myopathy occurs in the context of ACM, genetic causes readily explain these conditions, since some genes expressed in skeletal muscle also encode an important component of cardiac muscle. In addition to *LMNA*, noted previously, one should consider pathogenic variants in *DES* encoding desmin. Abnormalities in this gene associate with myofibrillar myopathy, occurring with ACM involving the left,

right, or both ventricles. Prominent founder mutations occur in the Netherlands, with lower prevalence throughout Europe and North America.[52,53] *FLNC* is another gene in which mutations were initially reported to cause myofibrillar myopathy, sometimes with cardiac involvement.[54] Analyses of larger cohorts with nonischemic cardiomyopathy included this gene on their panels.[55,56] This led to greater attention to the frequent arrhythmias occurring in families with pathogenic variants in *FLNC*, and more recently a report ties *FLNC* to ARVC.[57]

Two general themes are listed above, whereby mutations in genes encoding elements of the cell adhesion complexes or the nuclear envelope cause ACM. Another theme underlying the genetic basis of this form of cardiomyopathy arises from molecular chaperone proteins in the heart. *BAG3* encodes Bcl2-associated athanogene 3, which regulates cardiac contractility and calcium homeostasis, and pathogenic variants cause ACM.[58–60] Similarly, *RBM20* encodes an RNA-binding protein, which regulates splicing of many sarcomeric and calcium-handling genes.[61] Initial reports for pathogenic variants in *RBM20* identified its role in causing dilated cardiomyopathy.[62] Subsequently, several groups reported the arrhythmic tendency for families with abnormalities in this particular gene.[63,64] The most recent report cites high prevalence of family history of SCD (51%), as well as personal high prevalence of arrhythmias (43%) among affected individuals with *RBM20*-associated ACM.[64]

Limited data support genetic variation in the regulatory regions of *TGFB3* in association with ARVC. One report highlighted 2 families by genome-wide association analysis.[14] One of them had a variant in the 5′ untranslated region of this gene, and the other had a variant in the 3′ untranslated region.[65] Both variants associate with higher levels of *TGFB3* mRNA using an in vitro reporter protocol.[65]

Although rare, both variants are present in population databases. Other large studies did not identify rare variants in this gene associated with ACM, although loss-of-function variants in *TGFB3* do cause Loeys-Dietz syndrome, a disorder of aortic aneurysms and arterial tortuosity with systemic manifestations.[66] Without demonstration of increased *TGFB3* expression in tissues derived from individuals with these regulatory variants, and without additional support for the hypothesis that elevated expression of this gene causes ARVC, the significance of regulatory variants in *TGFB3* remains uncertain.

Whole Exome Sequencing Studies

In contrast with candidate-gene studies, whole exome sequencing (WES) analysis provides the opportunity for an unbiased platform from which to assess larger numbers of genes for their role in ACM. Several groups have utilized this approach to ascertain the genetic contributions to ACM among remaining probands and families without discernible pathogenic variants in genes with established ties to this phenotype. For instance, WES identified a rare variant in *SCN5A*, and further analysis showed that this variant causes reduced peak sodium current.[67] That led to testing a larger ACM cohort for pathogenic variants in *SCN5A*, with 5 (N = 281; 1.8%) having a convincing variant in this gene.[67] A similar approach for WES in 2 first cousins with ACM in South Africa identified approximately 13,000 heterozygous variants shared by both individuals.[68] After filtering for nonsynonymous variants with MAF ≤ 0.0001, 13 remained in consideration. Analysis in more affected family members helped to exclude some of these, and functional predictions focused on *CDH2*, encoding N-cadherin. Testing in a larger cohort of 73 unrelated South African probands with ARVC identified a second rare variant in this gene

with putative pathogenicity.[68] Another group subsequently validated this gene and this second rare variant by reporting its association with ARVC in another small family, similarly identified by WES.[69]

Collaboration between 2 European groups using WES also identified pathogenic variants in *TJP1*, which encodes ZO-1, a scaffolding protein involved with the cardiac intercalated disks.[70] Although determination of the true prevalence of mutations in this gene among families with ACM requires larger studies, this report identified rare variants in *TJP1* that were considered pathogenic in 4/84 (4.8%) unrelated probands.[70] This gene is rated highly for intolerance of loss-of-function variants (pLI = 1), with the prevalence of all putatively pathogenic variants having MAF < 0.01% only 0.19% in gnomAD.[70] Using similar analyses, WES also identified rare variants in *ILK*, which encodes integrin-linked kinase, as causing ACM in 2 unrelated families.[71]

Although WES can be used as an unbiased survey of the coding regions of all nuclear genes, it can also be used as an adjunct for comprehensive analysis in studies investigating novel genetic etiologies. Starting with an ACM proband who had clinical genetic testing with a platform of cardiomyopathy and arrhythmia genes, Roberts and colleagues identified an *ANK2* variant, which was previously linked to Ankyrin-B syndrome.[72,73] This focused the WES in another family, and identified a second putatively pathogenic variant in *ANK2*. Extension into a cohort of 207 unrelated probands with ARVC without a known gene mutation yielded 14 rare variants in *ANK2*.[73]

WES casts a very broad net when investigating small cohorts or families with ACM. This can lead to identification of promising rare variants, but it requires thorough analysis to conclude a pathogenic role. Some promising candidates fail this test. For instance, WES identified rare and putatively pathogenic variants in *SCN10A*, a gene that was previously associated with development of atrial fibrillation (AF) and Brugada syndrome.[74] Despite a constellation of rare variants in a cohort with unexplained ARVC, a similar frequency of rare variants also occurs among probands with ARVC and a desmosome gene mutation. The prevalence of rare variants in *SCN10A* was also quite similar among healthy Caucasian controls, leading to the conclusion that there is no primary role for *SCN10A* mutations in ARVC.[74] *PLEC* is another gene with very promising data by initial WES analysis.[75] This gene encodes plectin, a desmosome-associated cytolinker protein. Investigation of 3 separate ARVC cohorts identified one or more rare *PLEC* variants in 40/359 (11%) unrelated probands, which was similar between those with and without pathogenic/likely pathogenic desmosome gene variants.[75] Additionally, the prevalence of rare variants in PLEC was not higher among probands with ARVC than among control populations with 18% rare *PLEC* variants, supporting the conclusion of no major role for rare plectin variants in ARVC.[75]

The low cost and high throughput for next-generation DNA sequencing permits testing of large panels of genes for people with ACM. Because pathogenic variants in genes encoding elements of the cardiac sarcomere cause dilated, hypertrophic, and restrictive forms of cardiomyopathy, they are inevitably on these panels. In contrast with many other genes associated with ACM, pathogenic variants in sarcomere genes do not typically impart a high rate of arrhythmia, and their association with ACM is questionable. Among a cohort of 137 probands with ARVC without pathogenic variants in *PKP2*, *DSG2*, *DSP*, *DSC2*, *JUP*, *TMEM43*, *SCN5A*, and *PLN*, a collaborative study reported that 6 (4%) carried rare variants in 3 cardiac sarcomere genes: *MYH7*, *MYBPC3*, and *MYL3*.[76] The variants all had low prevalence in controls and were predicted to be damaging. However, segregation data in their small families were not informative, and the authors identified no clear mechanism for these variants to cause an isolated right ventricular (RV) cardiomyopathy or prominent arrhythmia. At this time, rare variants in sarcomere genes are unlikely to cause ACM.[76]

Reduced Penetrance

Despite classification as a Mendelian disorder, several groups have shown that ACM has low penetrance. Within families segregating ARVC and desmosome gene mutations, approximately one-third of family members meet TFC for this disorder, one-third of family members have phenotypic features without meeting the diagnostic threshold, and one-third have no discernible cardiac manifestations.[77,78] As with most inherited diseases, both genetic and environmental modifiers probably contribute. In the largest series of published patients with this condition, 4% of probands had more than one pathogenic variant contributing to their condition.[79] This supports a role for rare minor variants contributing to disease expression. Exercise is also a prominent factor in the pathogenesis of ACM, as explained in other sections of the proceedings from this meeting.[80] Autoimmunity and inflammation are also likely to be strong contributors to the penetrance and severity of ACM, as reviewed elsewhere in these proceedings.[81]

Relevance of Genetic Testing

Because genetic testing is now readily available and much lower in cost than in the past, its use has become much more common in clinical practice. As with other forms of inherited cardiovascular disease, there are several reasons to consider genetic testing. Although the presence of a pathogenic variant in an associated gene counts as a major criterion for the diagnosis of ARVC in the Revised TFC, most experts agree that use of genetic testing in probands is best performed with an unequivocal diagnosis.[82,83] Recognition of a DNA variant of uncertain significance in someone with an unclear phenotype does not lead to greater clarity. Use of genetic testing to achieve diagnostic criteria for ARVC or ACM in someone with an uncertain phenotype is controversial and discouraged by many experts.[84]

On the other hand, recognition of a pathogenic variant in an ACM proband facilitates the assessment of risk for ACM among family members. This can also be helpful for family planning. When used properly, the patient is informed about the potential outcomes of genetic testing, the likely costs, and the inherent risks, including the possibility of "genetic guilt."[85] Counseling by a trained genetic counselor should be provided, ideally both before and after the testing is performed. This should promote cascade genetic screening for ACM risk within families, and targeted phenotypic screening.

Genetic testing, genetic counseling, and variant interpretation should be performed in expert centers, as many challenges affect this evolving field. To address the complexity of genetic variation in human diseases, clinical laboratories and scientists around the world align data in a freely accessible public archive, called ClinVar. Ongoing curation efforts seek to improve the data in a collaboration called ClinGen.[86] Unfortunately, the relevance of most genes in which pathogenic variants are published in association with ACM have insufficient evidence for a definitive classification. Additionally, more than 10% of previously published pathogenic variants are classified as uncertain after closer review.[87] With time and greater scrutiny, as well as improved understanding of human genetic variation in different populations, the interpretation of rare DNA variants in ACM-associated genes should continue to improve.

Summary and Future Directions

Many genes are now associated with ACM, and specifically with the subset of ACM called ARVC. Pathogenic variants in genes encoding elements of the cardiac desmosome are the largest genetic contributors to this condition in most cohorts. Certain unique populations around the world have additional influence from prominent founder mutations. In the past few years, most additional genes tied to ACM explain a very small percentage (< 2%) of affected probands, and more than one-third of affected probands still do not have a clear genetic explanation for their condition. Noncoding variants, such as deep intronic nucleotide substitutions that alter exon splicing, are probably contributing, and they are difficult to identify. Future studies involving RNA sequencing and whole genome analysis may lead to better understanding of the depth and breadth of genetic contributions to ACM.

References

1. Marcus FI, Fontaine GH, Guiraudon G, Frank R, Laurenceau JL, Malergue C, Grosgogeat Y. Right ventricular dysplasia: A report of 24 adult cases. *Circulation.* 1982;65:384–398.

2. Ruder MA, Winston SA, Davis JC, Abbott JA, Eldar M, Scheinman MM. Arrhythmogenic right ventricular dysplasia in a family. *Am J Cardiol.* 1985;56:799–800.

3. Protonotarios N, Tsatsopoulou A, Patsourakos P, Alexopoulos D, Gezerlis P, Simitsis S, Scampardonis G. Cardiac abnormalities in familial palmoplantar keratosis. *Br Heart J.* 1986;56:321–326.

4. Coonar AS, Protonotarios N, Tsatsopoulou A, et al. Gene for arrhythmogenic right ventricular cardiomyopathy with diffuse nonepidermolytic palmoplantar keratoderma and woolly hair (Naxos disease) maps to 17q21. *Circulation.* 1998;97:2049–2058.

5. McKoy G, Protonotarios N, Crosby A, et al. Identification of a deletion in plakoglobin in arrhythmogenic right ventricular cardiomyopathy with palmoplantar keratoderma and woolly hair (Naxos disease). *Lancet.* 2000;355:2119–2124.

6. Carvajal-Huerta L. Epidermolytic palmoplantar keratoderma with woolly hair and dilated cardiomyopathy. *J Am Acad Dermatol.* 1998;39:418–421.

7. Norgett EE, Hatsell SJ, Carvajal-Huerta L, et al. Recessive mutation in desmoplakin disrupts desmoplakin-intermediate filament interactions and causes dilated cardiomyopathy, woolly hair and keratoderma. *Hum Mol Genet.* 2000;9:2761–2766.

8. Rampazzo A, Nava A, Danieli GA, et al. The gene for arrhythmogenic right ventricular cardiomyopathy maps to chromosome 14q23–q24. *Hum Mol Genet.* 1994;3:959–962.

9. Rampazzo A, Nava A, Erne P, et al. A new locus for arrhythmogenic right ventricular cardiomyopathy (ARVD2) maps to chromosome 1q42–q43. *Hum Mol Genet.* 1995;4:2151–2154.

10. Severini GM, Krajinovic M, Pinamonti B, et al. A new locus for arrhythmogenic right ventricular dysplasia on the long arm of chromosome 14. *Genomics.* 1996;31:193–200.

11. Rampazzo A, Nava A, Miorin M, et al. ARVD4, a new locus for arrhythmogenic right ventricular cardiomyopathy, maps to chromosome 2 long arm. *Genomics.* 1997;45:259–263.

12. Li D, Ahmad F, Gardner MJ, et al. The locus of a novel gene responsible for arrhythmogenic right-ventricular dysplasia characterized by early onset and high penetrance maps to chromosome 10p12–p14. *Am J Hum Genet.* 2000;66:148–156.

13. Melberg A, Oldfors A, Blomström-Lundqvist C, et al. Autosomal dominant myofibrillar myopathy with arrhythmogenic right ventricular cardiomyopathy linked to chromosome 10q. *Ann Neurol.* 1999;46:684–692.

14. Rampazzo A, Beffagna G, Nava A, et al. Arrhythmogenic right ventricular cardiomyopathy type 1 (ARVD1): Confirmation of locus assignment and mutation screening of four candidate genes. *Euro J Hum Genet.* 2003;11:69–76.

15. Rampazzo A, Nava A, Malacrida S, et al. Mutation in human desmoplakin domain binding to plakoglobin causes a dominant form of arrhythmogenic right ventricular cardiomyopathy. *Am J Hum Genet.* 2002;71:1200–1206.

16. Bauce B, Basso C, Rampazzo A, et al. Clinical profile of four families with arrhythmogenic right ventricular cardiomyopathy caused by dominant desmoplakin mutations. *Eur Heart J.* 2005;26:1666–1675.

17. Gerull B, Heuser A, Wichter T, et al. Mutations in the desmosomal protein plakophilin-2 are common in arrhythmogenic right ventricular cardiomyopathy. *Nat Genet.* 2004;36:1162–1164.

18. Grossmann KS, Grund C, Huelsken J, Behrend M, Erdmann B, Franke WW, Birchmeier W. Requirement of plakophilin 2 for heart morphogenesis and cardiac junction formation. *J Cell Biol.* 2004;167:149–160.

19. Christensen AH, Kamstrup PR, Gandjbakhch E, et al. Plakophilin-2 c.419C>T and risk of heart failure and arrhythmias in the general population. *Eur J Hum Genet.* 2016;24:732–738.

20. van Tintelen JP, Entius MM, Bhuiyan ZA, et al. Plakophilin-2 mutations are the major determinant of familial arrhythmogenic right ventricular dysplasia/cardiomyopathy. *Circulation.* 2006;113:1650–1658.

21. Dalal D, Molin LH, Piccini JP, et al. Clinical features of arrhythmogenic right ventricular dysplasia/cardiomyopathy associated with mutations in plakophilin-2. *Circulation.* 2006;113:1641–1649.

22. Syrris P, Ward D, Asimaki A, et al. Clinical expression of plakophilin-2 mutations in familial arrhythmogenic right ventricular cardiomyopathy. *Circulation.* 2006;113:356–364.

23. Hofmann I, Schlechter T, Kuhn C, Hergt M, Franke WW. Protein p0071: An armadillo plaque protein that characterizes a specific subtype of adherens junctions. *J Cell Sci.* 2009;122:21–24.

24. Chen X, Bonné S, Hatzfeld M, van Roy F, Green KJ. Protein binding and functional

characterization of plakophilin 2: Evidence for its diverse roles in desmosomes and β-catenin signaling. *J Biol Chem.* 2002;277:10512–10522.

25. Awad MM, Dalal D, Cho E, et al. DSG2 mutations contribute to arrhythmogenic right ventricular dysplasia/cardiomyopathy. *Am J Hum Genet.* 2006;79:136–142.

26. Pilichou K, Nava A, Basso C, et al. Mutations in desmoglein-2 gene are associated with arrhythmogenic right ventricular cardiomyopathy. *Circulation.* 2006;113:1171–1179.

27. Schäfer S, Koch PJ, Franke WW. Identification of the ubiquitous human desmoglein, Dsg2, and the expression catalogue of the desmoglein subfamily of desmosomal cadherins. *Exp Cell Res.* 1994;211:391–399.

28. Heuser A, Plovie ER, Ellinor PT, et al. Mutant desmocollin-2 causes arrhythmogenic right ventricular cardiomyopathy. *Am J Hum Genet.* 2006;79:1081–1088.

29. Syrris P, Ward D, Evans A, Asimaki A, Gandjbakhch E, Sen-Chowdhry S, McKenna WJ. Arrhythmogenic right ventricular dysplasia/cardiomyopathy associated with mutations in the desmosomal gene desmocollin-2. *Am J Hum Genet.* 2006;79:978–984.

30. Asimaki A, Syrris P, Wichter T, Matthias P, Saffitz JE, McKenna WJ. A novel fominant mutation in plakoglobin causes arrhythmogenic right ventricular cardiomyopathy. *Am J Hum Genet.* 2007;81:964–973.

31. van Lint FHM, Murray B, Tichnell C, et al. Arrhythmogenic right ventricular cardiomyopathy-associated desmosomal variants are rarely de novo. *Circ Genom Precis Med.* 2019;12:e002467.

32. Chen L, Rao M, Chen X, et al. A founder homozygous DSG2 variant in East Asia results in ARVC with full penetrance and heart failure phenotype. *Int J Cardiol.* 2019;274:263–270.

33. Franke WW, Borrmann CM, Grund C, Pieperhoff S. The area composita of adhering junctions connecting heart muscle cells of vertebrates. I. Molecular definition in intercalated disks of cardiomyocytes by immunoelectron microscopy of desmosomal proteins. *Eur J Cell Biol.* 2006;85:69–82.

34. van Hengel J, Calore M, Bauce B, et al. Mutations in the area composita protein alphaT-catenin are associated with arrhythmogenic right ventricular cardiomyopathy. *Eur Heart J.* 2013;34:201–210.

35. Marshall WH, Furey M, Larsen B, et al. Right ventricular cardiomyopathy and sudden death in young people. *N Engl J Med.* 1988;319:174–176.

36. Ahmad F, Li D, Karibe A, et al. Localization of a gene responsible for arrhythmogenic right ventricular dysplasia to chromosome 3p23. *Circulation.* 1998;98:2791–2795.

37. Hodgkinson KA, Parfrey PS, Bassett AS, et al. The impact of implantable cardioverter-defibrillator therapy on survival in autosomal-dominant arrhythmogenic right ventricular cardiomyopathy (ARVD5). *J Am Coll Cardiol.* 2005;45:400–408.

38. Merner ND, Hodgkinson KA, Haywood AFM, et al. Arrhythmogenic right ventricular cardiomyopathy type 5 is a fully penetrant, lethal arrhythmic disorder caused by a missense mutation in the TMEM43 gene. *Am J Hum Genet.* 2008;82:809–821.

39. Milting H, Klauke B, Christensen AH, et al. The TMEM43 Newfoundland mutation p.S358L causing ARVC-5 was imported from Europe and increases the stiffness of the cell nucleus. *Eur Heart J.* 2014;36:872–881.

40. Dominguez F, Zorio E, Jimenez-Jaimez J, et al. Clinical characteristics and determinants of the phenotype in TMEM43 arrhythmogenic right ventricular cardiomyopathy type 5. *Heart Rhythm.* 2020;17:945–954.

41. Meinke P, Nguyen TD, Wehnert MS. The LINC complex and human disease. *Biochem Soc Trans.* 2011;39:1693–1697.

42. van Tintelen JP, Hofstra RMW, Katerberg H, et al. High yield of LMNA mutations in patients with dilated cardiomyopathy and/or conduction disease referred to cardiogenetics outpatient clinics. *Am Heart J.* 2007;154:1130–1139.

43. Quarta G, Syrris P, Ashworth M, et al. Mutations in the Lamin A/C gene mimic arrhythmogenic right ventricular cardiomyopathy. *Eur Heart J.* 2012;33:1128–1136.

44. Abdelfatah N, Chen R, Duff HJ, et al. Characterization of a unique form of arrhythmic cardiomyopathy caused by recessive mutation in LEMD2. *JACC: Basic Translat Sci.* 2019;4:204–221.

45. Boone PM, Yuan B, Gu S, et al. Hutterite-type cataract maps to chromosome 6p21.32–p21.31, cosegregates with a homozygous mutation in LEMD2, and is associated with sudden cardiac death. *Mol Genet Genom Med.* 2016;4:77–94.

46. Tiso N, Stephan DA, Nava A, et al. Identification of mutations in the cardiac ryanodine receptor gene in families affected with arrhythmogenic right ventricular cardiomyopathy type 2 (ARVD2). *Hum Mol Genet.* 2001;10:189–194.

47. Priori SG, Napolitano C, Tiso N, et al. Mutations in the cardiac ryanodine receptor gene (hRyR2) underlie catecholaminergic polymorphic ventricular tachycardia. *Circulation.* 2001;103:196–200.

48. Haghighi K, Kolokathis F, Gramolini AO, et al. A mutation in the human phospholamban gene, deleting arginine 14, results in lethal, hereditary cardiomyopathy. *Proc Natl Acad Sci.* 2006;103:1388–1393.

49. Haghighi K, Kolokathis F, Pater L, et al. Human phospholamban null results in lethal dilated cardiomyopathy revealing a critical difference between mouse and human. *J Clin Invest.* 2003;111:869–876.

50. Schmitt JP, Kamisago M, Asahi M, et al. Dilated cardiomyopathy and heart failure caused by a mutation in phospholamban. *Science.* 2003;299:1410–1413.

51. van der Zwaag PA, van Rijsingen IAW, Asimaki A, et al. Phospholamban R14del mutation in patients diagnosed with dilated cardiomyopathy or arrhythmogenic right ventricular cardiomyopathy: Evidence supporting the concept of arrhythmogenic cardiomyopathy. *Eur J Heart Fail.* 2012;14:1199–1207.

52. van Spaendonck-Zwarts KY, van der Kooi AJ, van den Berg MP, et al. Recurrent and founder mutations in the Netherlands: The cardiac phenotype of DES founder mutations p.S13F and p.N342D. *Netherl Heart J.* 2012;20:219–228.

53. Lorenzon A, Beffagna G, Bauce B, et al. Desmin mutations and arrhythmogenic right ventricular cardiomyopathy. *Am J Cardiol.* 2013;111:400–405.

54. Ortiz-Genga MF, Cuenca S, Dal Ferro M, et al. Truncating FLNC mutations are associated with high-risk dilated and arrhythmogenic cardiomyopathies. *J Am Coll Cardiol.* 2016;68:2440–2451.

55. Begay RL, Graw SL, Sinagra G, et al. Filamin C truncation mutations are associated with arrhythmogenic dilated cardiomyopathy and changes in the cell–cell adhesion structures. *JACC: Clin Electrophysiol.* 2018;4:504–514.

56. Hall CL, Akhtar MM, Sabater-Molina M, et al. Filamin C variants are associated with a distinctive clinical and immunohistochemical arrhythmogenic cardiomyopathy phenotype. *Int J Cardiol.* 2019;307:101–108.

57. Brun F, Gigli M, Graw SL, Judge DP, et al. FLNC truncations cause arrhythmogenic right ventricular cardiomyopathy. *J Med Genet.* 2020:jmedgenet-2019-106394.

58. Feldman AM, Gordon J, Wang J, et al. BAG3 regulates contractility and Ca2+ homeostasis in adult mouse ventricular myocytes. *J Mol Cell Cardiol* 2016;92:10–20.

59. Norton N, Li D, Rieder Mark J, et al. Genome-wide studies of copy number variation and exome sequencing identify rare variants in BAG3 as a cause of dilated cardiomyopathy. *Am J Hum Genet.* 2011;88:273–282.

60. Domínguez F, Cuenca S, Bilińska Z, et al. Dilated cardiomyopathy due to BLC2-associated athanogene 3 (BAG3) mutations. *J Am Coll Cardiol.* 2018;72:2471–2481.

61. Maatz H, Jens M, Liss M, et al. RNA-binding protein RBM20 represses splicing to orchestrate cardiac pre-mRNA processing. *J Clin Invest.* 2014;124:3419–3430.

62. Brauch KM, Karst ML, Herron KJ, et al. Mutations in ribonucleic acid binding protein gene cause familial dilated cardiomyopathy. *J Am Coll Cardiol.* 2009;54:930–941.

63. Hoogenhof MMGvd, Beqqali A, Amin AS, et al. RBM20 mutations induce an arrhythmogenic dilated cardiomyopathy related to

disturbed calcium handling. *Circulation.* 2018;138:1330–1342.

64. Parikh VN, Caleshu C, Reuter C, et al. Regional variation in RBM20 causes a highly penetrant arrhythmogenic cardiomyopathy. *Circ Heart Fail.* 2019;12:e005371.

65. Beffagna G, Occhi G, Nava A, et al. Regulatory mutations in transforming growth factor-[beta]3 gene cause arrhythmogenic right ventricular cardiomyopathy type 1. *Cardiovasc Res.* 2005;65:366–373.

66. Bertoli-Avella AM, Gillis E, Morisaki H, et al. Mutations in a TGF-β ligand, TGFB3, cause syndromic aortic aneurysms and dissections. *J Am Coll Cardiol.* 2015;65:1324–1336.

67. te Riele ASJM, Agullo-Pascual E, James CA, et al. Multilevel analyses of SCN5A mutations in arrhythmogenic right ventricular dysplasia/cardiomyopathy suggest non-canonical mechanisms for disease pathogenesis. *Cardiovasc Res.* 2017;113:102–111.

68. Mayosi BM, Fish M, Shaboodien G, et al. Identification of cadherin 2 (CDH2) mutations in arrhythmogenic right ventricular cardiomyopathy. *Circ Cardiovasc Genet.* 2017;10:e001605.

69. Turkowski KL, Tester DJ, Bos JM, Haugaa KH, Ackerman MJ. Whole exome sequencing with genomic triangulation implicates CDH2-encoded N-cadherin as a novel pathogenic substrate for arrhythmogenic cardiomyopathy. *Congen Heart Dis.* 2017;12:226–235.

70. De Bortoli M, Postma AV, Poloni G, et al. Whole-exome sequencing identifies pathogenic variants in TJP1 gene associated with arrhythmogenic cardiomyopathy. *Circ Genom Precis Med.* 2018;11:e002123.

71. Brodehl A, Rezazadeh S, Williams T, et al. Mutations in ILK, encoding integrin-linked kinase, are associated with arrhythmogenic cardiomyopathy. *Transl Res.* 2019;208:15–29.

72. Mohler PJ, Schott J-J, Gramolini AO, et al. Ankyrin-B mutation causes type 4 long-QT cardiac arrhythmia and sudden cardiac death. *Nature.* 2003;421:634–639.

73. Roberts JD, Murphy NP, Hamilton RM, et al. Ankyrin-B dysfunction predisposes to arrhythmogenic cardiomyopathy and is amenable to therapy. *J Clin Invest.* 2019;129:3171–3184.

74. te Riele ASJM, James CA, Murray B, et al. Absence of a primary role for SCN10A mutations in arrhythmogenic right ventricular dysplasia/cardiomyopathy. *J Cardiovasc Transl Res.* 2016;9:87–89.

75. Hoorntje ET, Posafalvi A, Syrris P, et al. No major role for rare plectin variants in arrhythmogenic right ventricular cardiomyopathy. *PLoS One.* 2018;13:e0203078.

76. Murray B, Hoorntje ET, te Riele ASJM, et al. Identification of sarcomeric variants in probands with a clinical diagnosis of arrhythmogenic right ventricular cardiomyopathy (ARVC). *J Cardiovasc Electrophysiol.* 2018;29:1004–1009.

77. Dalal D, James C, Devanagondi R, et al. Penetrance of mutations in plakophilin-2 among families with arrhythmogenic right ventricular dysplasia/cardiomyopathy. *J Am Coll Cardiol.* 2006;48:1416–1424.

78. Quarta G, Muir A, Pantazis A, et al. Familial evaluation in arrhythmogenic right ventricular cardiomyopathy. *Circulation.* 2011;123: 2701–2709.

79. Groeneweg JA, Bhonsale A, James CA, et al. Clinical presentation, long-term follow-up, and outcomes of 1001 arrhythmogenic right ventricular dysplasia/cardiomyopathy patients and family members. *Circ Cardiovasc Genet.* 2015;8:437–446.

80. James CA, Bhonsale A, Tichnell C, et al. Exercise increases age-related penetrance and arrhythmic risk in arrhythmogenic right ventricular dysplasia/cardiomyopathy–associated desmosomal mutation Carriers. *J Am Coll Cardiol.* 2013;62:1290–1297.

81. Chatterjee D, Fatah M, Akdis D, et al. An autoantibody identifies arrhythmogenic right ventricular cardiomyopathy and participates in its pathogenesis. *Eur Heart J.* 2018;39:3932–3944.

82. Marcus FI, McKenna WJ, Sherrill D, et al. Diagnosis of arrhythmogenic right ventricular cardiomyopathy/dysplasia: Proposed modification of the Task Force Criteria. *Eur Heart J.* 2010;31:806–814.

83. Judge DP. Use of genetics in the clinical evaluation of cardiomyopathy. *JAMA*. 2009;302:2471–2476.

84. Corrado D, van Tintelen PJ, McKenna WJ, et al. Arrhythmogenic right ventricular cardiomyopathy: Evaluation of the current diagnostic criteria and differential diagnosis. *Eur Heart J*. 2019;41:1414–1429.

85. Kessler S, Kessler H, Ward P. Psychological aspects of genetic counseling. III. Management of guilt and shame. *Am J Med Genet*. 1984;17:673–697.

86. Rehm HL, Berg JS, Brooks LD, et al. ClinGen: The Clinical Genome Resource. *N Engl J Med*. 2015;372:2235–2242.

87. Ye JZ, Delmar M, Lundby A, Olesen MS. Reevaluation of genetic variants previously associated with arrhythmogenic right ventricular cardiomyopathy integrating population-based cohorts and proteomics data. *Clin Genet*. 2019;96:506–514.

7

Current Challenges in the Diagnosis of Arrhythmogenic Cardiomyopathies

Mimount Bourfiss, MD; Richard Hauer, MD, PhD

Introduction

Arrhythmogenic cardiomyopathies (ACMs) are a group of heart muscle diseases, usually hereditary, characterized histologically by ventricular fibrofatty alteration spreading from the subepicardium toward the subendocardium and clinically by ventricular arrhythmias (VAs) that usually start early in the disease process.[1-4] Although structural myocardial changes may occur in the early stage, hemodynamic dysfunction is usually an end-stage phenomenon. These characteristics distinguish ACM from dilated cardiomyopathy (DCM) with a different histology, early occurrence of heart failure, and usually ventricular and atrial arrhythmias at later stages.

Arrhythmogenic right ventricular dysplasia/cardiomyopathy (ARVD/C) or classical ARVC is the large subcategory of ACM with predominantly right ventricular (RV) involvement, described in the early 1980s by Fontaine and Marcus.[1] However, even in these early years, additional left ventricular (LV) involvement was observed in the end stage of disease. In more recent years, evidence of LV involvement in earlier disease stages at the molecular level has also been identified with immunofluorescence techniques.[5] Finally, balanced biventricular and predominant LV disease with similar histologic findings and early VA were discovered.[6] Recently, these observations supported the use of ACM as preferred nomenclature in an increasing number of publications. According to the most widely used definition of ACM, conditions without the typical fibrofatty alteration pattern are not included in this chapter on diagnosis. An alternative definition with a much wider disease spectrum and including also very different histologic patterns such as amyloidosis and Chagas disease has been proposed in a recent Heart Rhythm Society document.[7] However, that definition is not universally accepted and hence not chosen in this report.

The gold standard for ACM diagnosis is the fibrofatty alteration starting subepicardially and moving to the subendocardium.[4] This means that early in the disease process myocardial cell death and fibrofatty replacement are confined to subepicardial layers. Since fat is a physiologic phenomenon in the subepicardial area and more outspread in the so-called cor adiposum, differentiation from ACM may be difficult.[8] An incremental amount of fibrotic tissue and, if present, cell death are obligatory features for ACM diagnosis.[3,8] In more advanced stages, the typical histologic changes are frequently transmural in the thin-walled RV. Transmurality is rare in the LV. However, acquisition of appropriate histologic material by endomyocardial biopsy is hampered by the segmental nature of affected areas, usually absent involvement of interventricular septum and predominant subepicardial lesions early in the disease. Obviously, acquisition is easier during cardiac surgery, but only applicable at the end stage. These histologic limitations prompted the development of international consensus-based Task Force Criteria (TFC) for ARVC diagnosis in 1994, and revisions in 2010 (2010 TFC), as the surrogate gold standard.[9,10] These diagnostic TFC consist of a set of clinically available major and minor criteria in 6 categories (dysfunction and structural, histopathological, repolarization abnormalities, depolarization abnormalities, arrhythmias, and family history). At least 2 major, 1 major + 2 minor, or 4 minor TFC are required for fulfillment of ARVC diagnosis. In addition, ACM-mimicking disorders should be excluded. The 2010 TFC and methods for acquisition are illustrated in **Table 7.1**.[10] The 2010 TFC are a major improvement for classical ARVC diagnosis since they allow unequivocal diagnosis, facilitate comparison of studies, and are universally accepted.

However, the 2010 TFC also have limitations. With focus on the RV, 2010 TFC are less appropriate for LV involvement and inadequate for predominant LV disease. In addition, the focus in the RV is on the RV outflow tract (RVOT), which is open to criticism. Finally, weighing of electrocardiographic and genetic criteria should be reconsidered.

TABLE 7.1   Revised Task Force Criteria (2010)

Global and/or regional dysfunction and structural alterations (echo, MRI, cine-angio)
Tissue characterizations (histology from biopsy or autopsy)
Repolarization abnormalities (ECG)
Depolarization/conduction abnormalities (ECG, SAECG)
Arrythmias (ECG, Holter, exercise test)
Family history (ARVD/C in first-degree relative, pathogenic mutation)

ARVD/C diagnosis requires: 2 major criteria, 1 major + 2 minor, or 4 minor criteria, in the absence of other cause.

Diagnosis in Biventricular and Predominant LV Disease

Clinically relevant LV disease is unusual in classical ARVC, with the exception of the end stage (see **Figure 7.1**), which exhibits similar fibrofatty alteration in the RV and LV (**Figure 7.2**). RV predominance is very typical for ACM-associated desmosmal *PKP2* mutation carriers.[11-14] In many cohorts, *PKP2* is by far the most frequent molecular genetic abnormality in classical ARVC. Although ACM is frequently described as a disease of the desmosome, different desmosomal mutations may be associated with different disease patterns. The desmosomal *DSP* is associated with biventricular or even predominant LV disease (**Figure 7.3**), similar to the nondesmosomal *PLN* mutation.[13,15-19] Nevertheless, all these different disease entities show very similar fibrofatty alteration patterns, justifying ACM as unifying preferred terminology.[4]

In the 2010 TFC, only inverted T waves in the left precordial leads V_4–V_6 reflect LV involvement and only as a minor criterion.[10]

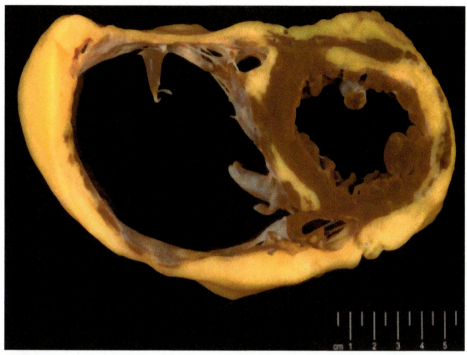

FIGURE 7.1 Slice of the explanted heart from a 56-year-old woman with end-stage ACM and the pathogenic missense mutation *PKP2* c.2386T>C. The RV is severely dilated, and the free wall is nearly completely transmurally replaced by fibrofatty tissue. In addition, there is extensive fibrofatty alteration in the LV and septum. The LV shows the typical predominant subepicardial involvement.

RV   LV

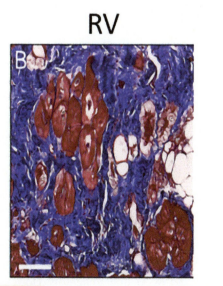
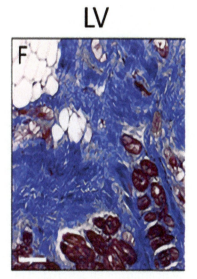

FIGURE 7.2 Histology from the heart in Figure 7.1 of the RV (**left panel**) and LV (**right panel**) shows similar fibrofatty alterations (modified AZAN staining). Surviving myocardial bundles are shown (**red**) embedded in fibrous tissue (**blue**) and fields of fat cells (**white**).

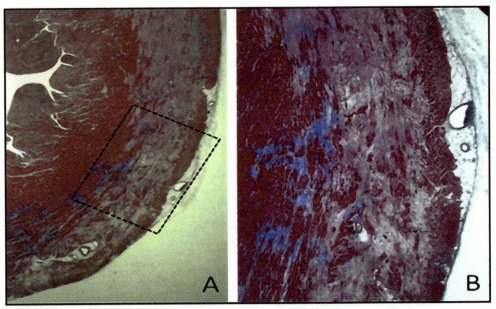

FIGURE 7.3 LV histology at two different magnifications from a 15-year-old sudden cardiac death victim with a pathogenic *DSP* mutation. In **Panel A**, the typical subepicardial involvement is visible. In **Panel B**, with more magnification, fibrofatty alterations are seen. The RV did not show obvious abnormality. Eight months before death, none of the 2010 TFC have been identified. (Figure reproduced with permission from Oxford University Press. Zorzi et al., *Europace*. 2016;18(7):1086–1094.[16])

In ACM with LV disease, the majority of electrocardiographic and imaging 2010 TFC may be absent, hampering diagnostic fulfillment. In addition, ACM patients with LV disease may not show ventricular tachycardia (VT) with left bundle branch block (LBBB) morphology. Different from classical ARVC, they may show VT with right bundle branch block (RBBB) morphology, reflecting the LV origin of the arrhythmia. However, RBBB-VT is not part of the 2010 TFC. Since ventricular mass is predominantly related to LV mass, and myocardial mass is related to QRS amplitude, low voltages in the electroocardiogram (ECG) during sinus rhythm are expected in late stages of LV disease.[20] Similarly, this larger LV mass precludes akinesia, dyskinesia, dilatation, and lowering of the ejection fraction in the earlier stages of LV disease with usually nontransmural lesions.[21] Thus, structural and hemodynamic dysfunction equivalents of ACM starting in the RV are not likely seen in the LV, at least in the earlier stages.

This means that the role of echocardiography and conventional cardiac magnetic resonance (CMR) is limited. Fortunately, the newer late gadolinium enhancement (LGE) technique during CMR, not used in the 2010 TFC scoring, is able to visualize smaller, nontransmural lesions reflecting fibrofatty areas.[21]

Thus, awareness of ACM as not only an RV disease but frequently also an LV disease and existence of even predominant LV subcategories prompt consideration of the following additional parameters for diagnostic evaluation:

- LGE-CMR to demonstrate LV lesions
- VT with RBBB morphology
- Low-voltage ECG (< 0.5 mV in standard leads during sinus rhythm)

Adding these parameters to the 2010 TFC will avoid ACM underdiagnosis. However, it should be realized that these parameters need confirmation and that their weight in relation to existing TFC is still unknown.

Electrocardiographic Challenges in ACM Diagnosis

In the 2010 TFC, the epsilon wave is a major criterion, since this finding is associated with advanced ACM. Comparing different studies, the incidence of epsilon waves varies between 2% in family members of ACM patients and 15% in index patients in the largest ACM study consisting of more than 1000 ACM patients and their family members, and much higher percentages in some other studies.[14] These differences may be due to differences in disease severity, but may also relate to the use of different definitions of the epsilon wave. Lower percentages are obtained by using the original definition by Fontaine et al. as low-amplitude signals after and clearly separated from the QRS complex in leads V_1–V_3.[22,23] Separation suggests the presence of an isoelectric line between the epsilon wave and the preceding QRS complex. However, identification of this isoelectric line depends on recording speed, filter setting, magnification, and sampling frequency. **Figure 7.4** shows an example of an ECG recorded from a patient with advanced ACM, negative T waves in V_1–V_5 (major repolarization criterion), prolonged terminal activation duration (TAD, 110 ms), and the suggestion of an epsilon wave (major depolarization criterion).[23] With 2 major criteria, this ECG already fulfills 2010 TFC for ACM diagnosis. However, separation from the QRS complex may be questioned, since very tiny signals are visible. Those who do not include the separation are faced with defining the end of the QRS complex and the onset of the epsilon wave. In a multicenter study by Platonov et al., epsilon wave identification showed

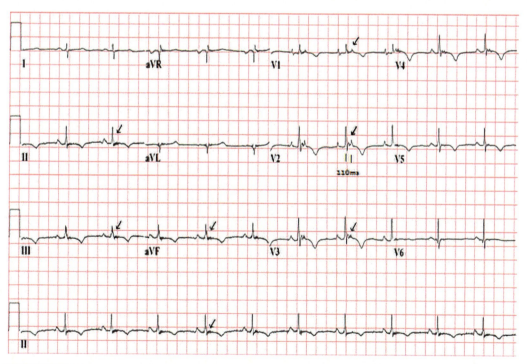

FIGURE 7.4 ECG during sinus rhythm from a patient with advanced ACM. Terminal activation duration is severely prolonged at 110 ms (minor criterion). The latest depolarization deflection indicated by **arrows** in V_1–V_3 may be interpreted as epsilon waves. However, tiny deflections are visible between this deflection and the preceding QRS complex. T-wave inversion in V_1–V_5 (major criterion). In addition, multiple late signals are present in inferior leads. (Reproduced with permission from Cardiotext Publishing, LLC.)

high interobserver variability.[24] In addition, all patients with interpretation of an epsilon wave had prolonged TAD (minor depolarization criterion) and showed ACM fulfillment independent of the epsilon wave.

Inverted T waves in the right precordial leads is much more common in athletes than in nonathletes in an apparently normal population.[25] Particularly with negative T waves in V_1–V_3 and beyond (major TFC criterion) and dilated RV, which can be found in normal athletes, differentiation with ACM may be difficult. Absence of abnormal depolarization and akinesia/dyskinesia support absence of ACM. In a recent study comparing 100 healthy athletes with 100 ACM patients, no premature ventricular complexes (PVCs) in the athletes and at least 1 PVC in 18 ACM patients ($P < 0.001$) were recorded during 10-second ECG recording. In addition, QRS voltages were significantly higher in the athletes.[26]

Both the depolarization criteria—epsilon wave and prolonged TAD ($\geq$ 55 ms)—and the repolarization criteria of inverted T wave in V_1–V_2 and V_1–V_3 and beyond focus on right precordial leads. That focus may be questioned. The right precordial leads reflect primarily electrical phenomena from the RVOT. However, the frequently recorded VT with LBBB morphology with superior axis (major arrhythmia TFC) is not originating from the RVOT.[10] The RVOT belongs to the "triangle of dysplasia" consisting of the 3 RV sites—the RVOT and subtricuspid and apical areas—most often affected in classical ARVC according to the original description of the disease in 1982.[1] This observation was primarily obtained from studying patients in advanced disease stages. A recent CMR study by te Riele et al. could confirm this observation if $\geq$ 3 RV regions were affected.[21] However, with only 1 or 2 affected regions, it was exclusively localized in the subtricuspid (or peritricuspid) area. This finding suggests disease onset close to the tricuspid valve and not in the RVOT or RV apex (**Figure 7.5**).

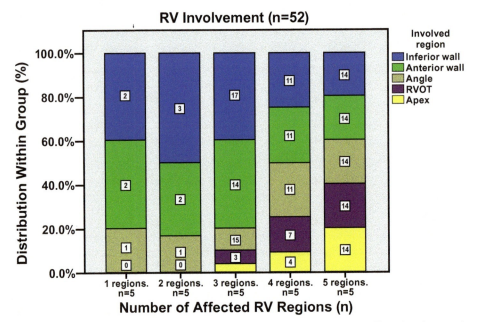

FIGURE 7.5   Number of affected RV regions in 52 ACM patients related to distribution of specific regions in percentages. If only 1 or 2 regions are affected, RV apex and RVOT are not involved. (Figure reproduced with permission from Wiley. te Riele et al., *J Cardiovasc Electrophysiol*. 2013;24:1311–1320.[21])

This finding is clinically relevant since it prompts us to identify subtricuspid disease markers for early disease detection. Under physiologic conditions, the RVOT is usually the latest activated area. Thus, additional pathological activation delay is relatively easily detectable in the RVOT and thus in right precordial leads by TAD prolongation.[23]

Physiologically, subtricuspid activation is usually earlier, indicating that local additional delay may remain buried within the QRS complex. Nevertheless, extreme delay may become visible as late activation mimicking precordial TAD but now recorded from the inferior leads (see **Figure 7.4**, **Figure 7.6**, and **Figure 7.7**).

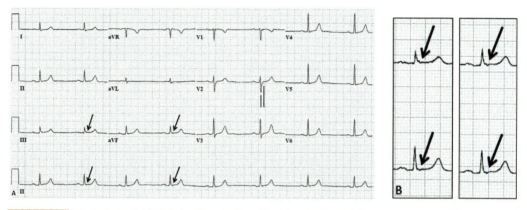

FIGURE 7.6 Apparently normal ECG during sinus rhythm, although terminal activation duration is marginally prolonged at 60 ms. However, very low amplitude but reproducible late depolarization signals are recorded in the inferior leads, enlarged in the **right panel**. (Reproduced with permission from Cardiotext Publishing, LLC.)

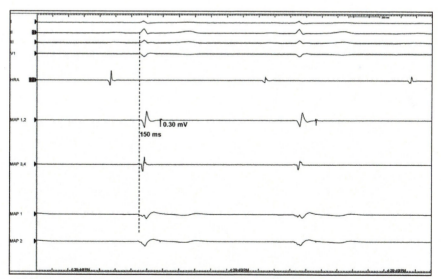

FIGURE 7.7 Electrophysiologic study during sinus rhythm in the patient from Figure 7.6. From above, ECG leads I, II, III, and V₁, bipolar recordings from the high right atrium, subtricuspid area (MAP 1,2 and MAP 3,4), and corresponding unipolar recordings MAP 1 and MAP 2 from tip and second electrode. The vertical line indicates the onset of the QRS complex. In MAP 1,2 a late 0.30 mV high dV/dt signal is recorded at 150 ms after QRS onset. The unipolar recording shows that this signal is derived from close to the position of electrode MAP 2 in the subtricuspid area. Earlier, higher-amplitude but lower dV/dt signals are from remote regions. (Reproduced with permission from Cardiotext Publishing, LLC.)

Recordings in Figure 7.4 are from a severely affected patient with 2 major electrocardiographic TFC from right precordial leads. In addition, late depolarization with multiple deflections and inverted T waves are recorded from the inferior leads. Figure 7.6 shows an apparently normal ECG in a patient with a pathogenic *PKP2* mutation. However, TAD is marginally at 60 ms prolonged, and with close observation, reproducibly isolated, late, low-amplitude signals are visible derived from the inferior leads. Remarkably, no inverted T waves are seen in this recording. An electrophysiologic study proved late depolarization as cause of these signals (Figure 7.7).[27] CMR showed a subtricuspid aneurysm in the absence of other pathologic markers (**Figure 7.8**).[27] Since in less advanced ACM stages, ECG signs of subtricuspid involvement remain invisible, other diagnostic techniques such as LGE-CMR, feature tracking CMR, and echocardiographic deformation imaging are promising for early ACM diagnosis.[28–30]

The last 2 techniques are based on delayed contraction, at least partly due to late electrical activation. **Figure 7.9** shows a normal 12-lead ECG without any sign of depolarization or repolarization abnormality. However, echocardiographic deformation imaging shows exclusively late contraction in the subtricuspid area (**Figure 7.10**).[28] Similar results are obtainable with feature tracking CMR.[30] More focus on the early affected subtricuspid area is clinically relevant since sudden cardiac death (SCD) is frequently the first ACM manifestation, particularly in young individuals as shown in several studies.[13,31–33]

One of these studies compared first presentation with ACM in 427 adults ≥18 years of age versus 75 pediatric patients < 18 years.[32] Combined SCD and resuscitated cardiac arrest in the adult and pediatric population occurred in 9% and 26%, respectively (**Figure 7.11**). In another study with 66 cardiac arrest cases in ACM, more than half of the victims appeared to be asymptomatic before

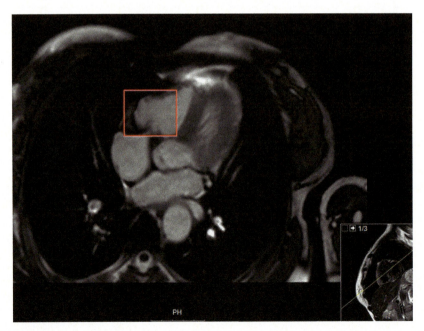

FIGURE 7.8 CMR image from the patient in Figures 7.6 and 7.7, showing a subtricuspid aneurysm. (Reproduced with permission from Cardiotext Publishing, LLC.)

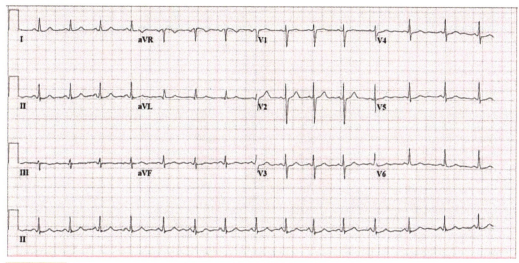

FIGURE 7.9 ECG from an asymptomatic pathogenic *PKP2* (c.397C>T) carrier. The ECG is normal and without depolarization or repolarization abnormalities. (Reproduced from *J Cardiovasc Electrophysiol.* 2016;27(3):303–314, with permission from Wiley.)

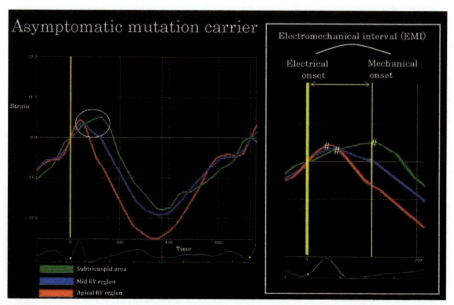

FIGURE 7.10 RV deformation imaging in the asymptomatic patient from Figure 7.9, magnified at the right side. Apical and midventricular curves are normal, whereas the subtricuspid area shows marked delayed contraction, at least partly due to local delayed electrical activation, not visible with the ECG. (Reproduced from *J Cardiovasc Electrophysiol.* 2016;27(3):303–314. with permission from Wiley.)

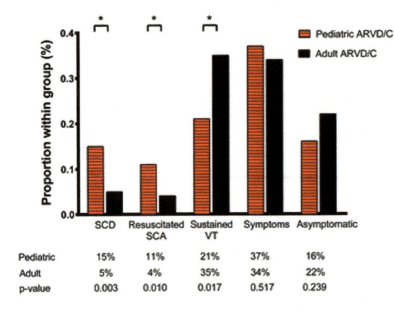

	SCD	Resuscitated SCA	Sustained VT	Symptoms	Asymptomatic
Pediatric	15%	11%	21%	37%	16%
Adult	5%	4%	35%	34%	22%
p-value	0.003	0.010	0.017	0.517	0.239

FIGURE 7.11 First presentation in ACM in adult (age ≥18 years, n = 475) versus pediatric (age < 18 years, n = 75) patients. SCD and resuscitated cardiac arrest are the first ACM manifestations in 9% of adult population and in the 26% of children. (Figure reproduced with permission from Elsevier. te Riele et al., *JACC Clin Electrophysiol.* 2015;1:551–560.[32])

this event.[33] In young individuals still in the early preclinical or concealed stages of ACM, fulfillment of diagnostic criteria may be absent. Ventricular fibrillation (VF) may be labeled as idiopathic VF and an implantable cardioverter-defibrillator (ICD) is implanted to prevent sudden death.[34] Beside ICD interrogation, regular cardiologic evaluation with at least family history, 12-lead ECG, and echocardiography is needed, and in some cases also additional DNA analysis.

Using this continuous evaluation ACM diagnostic fulfillment may occur many years after first presentation.[34] Definite diagnosis is important for cascade screening of family members as a first step in risk stratification.

Use of alternative diagnostic ECG methods such as signal-averaged ECG (SAECG, included in 2010 TFC) and QRS fractionation (fQRS) are hampered by several limitations.[35–38] Both methods are not universally used, and the use of SAECG for ACM diagnosis is decreasing. Moreover, late potentials recorded by SAECG are equivalents of easily obtained prolonged TAD in V_1–V_3 and late depolarization signals derived from other leads in the routine 12-lead ECG. Qualitative fQRS is prone to subjectivity and poor reproducibility between studies.[36–38] Quantitative methods for ACM diagnosis are not available yet.

Thus, contribution of the routine 12-lead ECG to ACM diagnosis is hampered by:

- Inaccuracy and nonreproducibility of epsilon wave recording.
- Although very appropriate in overt classic ARVC stages, less usefulness of precordial depolarization/repolarization abnormality detection in the early disease stage, because of evidence of early exclusive subtricuspid involvement.
- Absence of ECG detectability of subtricuspid involvement except in advanced stages, necessitating the use of new imaging techniques.
- ACM overdiagnosis by precordial T-wave inversion creating ACM phenocopies in athletes.

Genetic Challenges in ACM Diagnosis

The current 2010 TFC consist of 3 major and 3 minor genetic criteria.[10] Further weighting within the major and minor criteria is not available yet. A pathogenic or likely pathogenic mutation is counted as major criterion.

However, the high genetic noise due to frequent disease-associated genetic variants in the normal population and other cardiomyopathies are associated with the risk of misdiagnosis, particularly if the phenotype scoring reveals only 1 major or 2 minor criteria.[35,39] In addition, increasing genetic knowledge may devaluate a likely pathogenic variant to a variant of unknown significance. This means that results of molecular-genetic analysis should be interpreted by experts in the field. Since identification of a disease-causing mutation in the proband allows cascade screening in the family as a first step in their risk stratification, molecular-genetic analysis remains pivotal.[13,14]

Conclusion

Appropriate weighting of the contribution of each individual criterion of the 2010 TFC is still missing. Diagnostic challenges in ACM are in under- and overdiagnosis.

Underdiagnosis is related to (1) ignorance of LV and RV subtricuspid involvement and (2) paucity of criteria in early disease stage and young individuals. Inclusion of LGE-CMR and new imaging techniques such as echocardiographic deformation imaging and feature tracking CMR may contribute to improve the current TFC. Overdiagnosis relates to (1) inappropriate use of ECG and imaging criteria, (2) uncertainty about pathogenicity of gene variants, and (3) ACM phenocopies.

Devaluation of major criterion status of epsilon wave and likely pathogenicity may contribute to decrease of overdiagnosis.

References

1. Marcus FI, Fontaine GH, Guiraudon G, et al. Right ventricular dysplasia: A report of 24 adult cases. *Circulation.* 1982;65(2):384–398.
2. Corrado D, Basso C, Thiene G, et al. Spectrum of clinicopathologic manifestations of arrhythmogenic right ventricular cardiomyopathy/dysplasia: A multicenter study. *J Am Coll Cardiol.* 1997;30:1512–1520.
3. Basso C, Thiene G, Corrado D, et al. Arrhythmogenic right ventricular cardiomyopathy: Dysplasia, dystrophy, or myocarditis? *Circulation.* 1996;94:983–991.
4. Sepehrkhouy S, Gho J, van Es R, et al. Distinct fibrosis pattern in desmosomal and phospholamban mutation carriers in hereditary cardiomyopathies. *Heart Rhythm.* 2017;14:1024–1032.
5. Asimaki A, Tandri H, Huang H, et al. A new diagnostic test for arrhythmogenic right ventricular cardiomyopathy. *N Engl J Med.* 2009;360:1075–1064.
6. Sen-Chowdry S, Syrris P, Prasad SK, et al. Left-dominant arrhythmogenic cardiomyopathy: An under-recognized clinical entity. *J Am Coll Cardiol.* 2008;52:2175–2187.
7. Towbin JA, McKenna WJ, Abrams DJ, et al. 2019 HRS expert consensus statement on evaluation, risk stratification, and management of arrhythmogenic cardiomyopathy. *Heart Rhythm.* 2019;16(11):e301–e372.
8. Basso C, Thiene G. Adipositas cordis, fatty infiltration of the right ventricle, and arrhythmogenic right ventricular cardiomyopathy. Just a matter of fat? *Cardiovasc Pathol.* 2005;14(1):37–41.
9. McKenna WJ, Thiene G, Nava A, et al. Diagnosis of arrhythmogenic right ventricular dysplasia/cardiomyopathy. Task Force of the Working Group Myocardial and Pericardial Disease of the European Society of Cardiology and of the Scientific Council on Cardiomyopathies of the International Society and Federation of Cardiology. *Br Heart J.* 1994;71:215–218.
10. Marcus FI, McKenna WJ, Sherrill D, et al. Diagnosis of arrhythmogenic right ventricular cardiomyopathy/dysplasia: Proposed modification of the Task Force Criteria. *Eur Heart J.* 2010;31:806–814.
11. Van Tintelen JP, Entius MM, Bhuiyan ZA, et al. Plakophilin-2 mutations are the major determinant of familial arrhythmogenic right ventricular dysplasia/cardiomyopathy. *Circulation.* 2006;113:1650–1658.
12. Cox MG, van der Zwaag PA, van der Werf C, et al. Arrhythmogenic right ventricular dysplasia/cardiomyopathy: Pathogenic des-

mosome mutations in index-patients predict outcome of family screening: Dutch arrhythmogenic right ventricular dysplasia/cardiomyopathy genotype-phenotype follow-up study. *Circulation.* 2011;123:2690–2700.

13. Bhonsale A, Groeneweg JA, James CA, et al. Impact of genotype on clinical course in arrhythmogenic right ventricular dysplasia/cardiomyopathy-associated mutation carriers. *Eur Heart J.* 2015;36:847–855.

14. Groeneweg JA, Bhonsale A, James CA, et al. Clinical presentation, long-term follow-up, and outcomes of 1001 arrhythmogenic right ventricular dysplasia/cardiomyopathy patients and family members. *Circ Cardiovasc Genet.* 2015;8:437–446.

15. Norman M, Simpson M, Mogensen J, et al. Novel mutation in desmoplakin causes arrhythmogenic left ventricular cardiomyopathy. *Circulation.* 2005;112:636–642.

16. Zorzi A, Rigato I, Pilichou K, et al. Phenotypic expression is a prerequisite for malignant arrhtyhmic events and sudden cardiac death in arrhythmogenic right ventricular cardiomyopathy. *Europace.* 2016;18(7):1086–1094.

17. Van der Zwaag PA, van Rijsingen IA, Asimaki A, et al. Phospholamban R14del mutation in patients diagnosed with dilated cardiomyopathy or arrhythmogenic right ventricular cardiomyopathy: Evidence supporting the concept of arrhythmogenic cardiomyopathy. *Eur J Heart Fail.* 2012;14:1199–1207.

18. Groeneweg JA, van der Zwaag PA, Jongbloed JD, et al. Left-dominant arrhythmogenic cardiomyopathy in a large family: Associated desmosomal or nondesmosomal genotype? *Heart Rhythm.* 2013;10:548–559.

19. Groeneweg JA, van der Zwaag PA, Olde Nordkamp LR, et al. Arrhythmogenic right ventricular dysplasia/cardiomyopathy according to revised 2010 Task Force Criteria with inclusion of non-desmosomal phospholamban mutation carriers. *Am J Cardiol.* 2013;112:1197–206.

20. di Gioia CR, Giordano C, Cerbelli B, et al. Nonischemic left ventricular scar and cardiac sudden death in the young. *Hum Pathol.* 2016;58:78–89.

21. te Riele AS, James CA, Philips B, et al. Mutation-positive arrhythmogenic right ventricular dysplasia/cardiomyopathy: The triangle of dysplasia displaced. *J Cardiovasc Electrophysiol.* 2013;24:1311–1320.

22. Fontaine G, Umemura J, Di Donna P, et al. Duration of QRS complexes in arrhythmogenic right ventricular dysplasia-cardiomyopathy: A new non-invasive diagnostic marker. *Ann Cardiol Angeiol.* (Paris) 1993;42: 399–405.

23. Cox MGPJ, Nelen MR, Wilde AAM, et al. Activation delay and VT parameters in arrhythmogenic right ventricular dysplasia/cardiomyopathy toward improvement of diagnostic ECG criteria. *J Cardiovasc Electrophysiol.* 2008;19:775–781.

24. Platonov PG, Calkins H, Hauer RN, et al. High interobserver variability in the assessment of epsilon waves: Implications for diagnosis of arrhythmogenic right ventricular cardiomyopathy/dysplasia. *Heart Rhythm.* 2016;13:208–216.

25. Zaidi A, Sheikh N, Jongman JK, et al. Clinical differentiation between physiological remodeling and arrhythmogenic right ventricular cardiomyopathy in athletes with marked electrocardiographic repolarization anomalies. *J Am Coll Cardiol.* 2015;65:2702–2711.

26. Brosnan MJ, te Riele ASJM, Bosman LP, et al. Electrocardiographic features differentiating arrhythmogenic right ventricular cardiomyopathy from an athlete's heart. *JACC Clin Electrophysiol.* 2018;4(12):1626–1628.

27. ECG masters' collection, eds. Shenassa M, Josephson ME, Estes NA, Amsterdam EA, Scheinman M. 2017:461–463.

28. Mast TP, Teske AJ, te Riele ASJM, et al. Prolonged electromechanical interval unmasks arrhythmogenic right ventricular dysplasia/cardiomyopathy in the subclinical stage. *J Cardiovasc Electrophysiol.* 2016;27(3): 303–314.

29. Mast TP, James CA, Calkins H, et al. Evaluation of structural progression in arrhythmogenic right ventricular dysplasia/cardiomyopathy. *JAMA Cardiol.* 2017;2:293–302.

30. Bourfiss M, Vigneault DM, Aliyari Ghasebeh M, et al. Feature tracking CMR reveals abnormal strain in preclinical arrhythmogenic right ventricular dysplasia/cardiomyopathy: A multisoftware feasibility and clinical implementation study. *J Cardiovasc Magn Reson.* 2017;19(1):66. https://doi.org/10.1186/s12968-017-0380-4.

31. Quarta G, Muir A, Pantazis A, et al. Familial evaluation in arrhythmogenic right ventricular cardiomyopathy: Impact of genetics and revised Task Force Criteria. *Circulation.* 2011;123:2701–2709.

32. te Riele A, James CA, Sawant AC, et al. Arrhythmogenic right ventricular dysplasia/cardiomyopathy in the pediatric population: Clinical characterization and comparison with adult-onset disease. *JACC Clin Electrophysiol.* 2015;1:551–560.

33. Gupta R, Tichnell C, Murray B, et al. Comparison of features of fatal versus nonfatal cardiac arrest in patients with arrhythmogenic right ventricular dysplasia/cardiomyopathy. *Am J Cardiol.* 2017 Jul 1;120(1):111–117.

34. Blom LJ, te Riele ASJM, Vink A, et al. Late evolution of arrhythmogenic cardiomyopathy in patients with initial presentation as idiopathic ventricular fibrillation. *Heart Rhythm Case Rep.* 2019;5(1):25–30.

35. Corrado D, van Tintelen PJ, McKenna WJ, et al. Arrhythmogenic right ventricular cardiomyopathy: Evaluation of the current diagnostic criteria and differential diagnosis. *Eur Heart J.* 2019 Oct 21. pii: ehz669. doi:10.1093/eurheartj/ehz669 [Epub ahead of print].

36. Malik M. Electrocardiographic smoke signals of fragmented QRS complex. *J Cardiovasc Electrophysiol.* 2013;24:1267–1270.

37. Bosman LP, Sammani A, James CA, et al. Predicting arrhythmic risk in arrhythmogenic right ventricular cardiomyopathy: A systematic review and meta-analysis. *Heart Rhythm.* 2018;15:1097–1107.

38. Haukilahti MA, Eranti A, Kentta T, Huikuri HV. QRS fragmentation patterns representing myocardial scar need to be separated from benign normal variants: Hypotheses and proposal for morphology based classification. *Front Physiol.* 2016;7:653.

39. Kapplinger JD, Landstrom AP, Salisbury BA, et al. Distinguishing arrhythmogenic right ventricular cardiomyopathy/dysplasia-associated mutations from background genetic noise. *J Am Coll Cardiol.* 2011;57:2317–2327.

8

Differential Diagnosis of Phenotypic Variants of Arrhythmogenic Cardiomyopathy

Hugh Calkins, MD

Introduction

Arrhythmogenic right ventricular dysplasia/cardiomyopathy (ARVD/C) is an inherited cardiomyopathy that is characterized by ventricular arrhythmias (VAs), an increased risk of sudden death, and abnormalities of right (and less commonly left) ventricular structure and function. The first major description of this disease was published by Marcus et al. in 1982.[1] This paper described the clinical features of 22 patients with ventricular tachycardia (VT) who were diagnosed with right ventricular (RV) dysplasia. Key features of this condition were a dilated RV with wall motion abnormalities, particularly in the infundibulum. The paper notes the left ventricular (LV) diastolic size was normal. There are no other comments about LV size or function. It is worth noting that the imaging modalities were limited at that time and importantly did not include cardiac magnetic resonance imaging (MRI).

The perspective on ARVC as a right-dominant disease shifted in 2002, when Hamid and McKenna called for a need to broaden the diagnostic criteria.[2] In this landmark paper, 298 relatives of 67 probands diagnosed with ARVC were evaluated. Twenty-nine of these relatives had ARVC. LV involvement was present in 21% of these affected individuals.

Corrado et al. recently wrote an article that emphasized the fact that we are now keenly aware that ARVC can present as a right-dominant disease, as a left-dominant disease, or with involvement of both the RV and the LV.[3] In this article, the limitations of the 2010 diagnostic criteria were reviewed, and a proposal was made for new diagnostic criteria for the left-dominant or biventricular forms of the disease.

In 2019, the Heart Rhythm Society (HRS) published an expert consensus document on the evaluation, risk stratification, and management of arrhythmogenic cardiomyopathy.[4]

This document took a big-tent approach to the term *arrhythmogenic cardiomyopathy* (ACM). ACM was defined as a condition with VAs as a prominent part of the clinical presentation combined with structural heart disease, or, as Perry Elliot likes to state, ACM describes patients with a "twitchy heart."

In this chapter, we will review the differential diagnosis of ARVC and biventricular ALVC. We will also review some of the ways in which these conditions can be distinguished. Finally, we will provide a brief review of the HRS 2019 Consensus Document on ACM.

Differential Diagnosis of ARVC

Diagnosis of ARVC is challenging and is based on the 2010 diagnostic criteria.[5] Patients with suspected ARVC should undergo comprehensive testing, including a 12-lead electrocardiogram (ECG), Holter, and cardiac MRI (or ECG if an MRI cannot be performed). It is also essential to perform a family history. Genetic testing is generally reserved for patients who meet or almost meet diagnostic criteria.

When ARVC is suspected, a number of other conditions need to be included in the differential diagnosis. The importance of a broad differential diagnosis was recognized by Marcus and Fontaine in their landmark article in 1982.[1] In this article, they note that the differential diagnosis should include congenital anomalies such as an atrial septal defect, abnormal pulmonary venous return, congenital pulmonary regurgitation, pectus excavatum, Ebstein's anomaly, and congenital absence of the left pericardium. With time, it has become clear that the differential diagnosis of ARVC is even more extensive. **Table 8.1** shows the current differential diagnosis for ARVC.

Among the more challenging conditions to distinguish from ARVC are cardiac sarcoidosis and idiopathic VT. A large number of articles have been written that have called attention to the fact that it is not uncommon for patients with cardiac sarcoidosis to meet all of the diagnostic criteria for ARVC. Philips et al. compared the clinical features of 15 patients with cardiac sarcoidosis who met the diagnostic criteria for ARVC with those of 42 ARVC patients with a pathogenic mutation.[6] Patients with cardiac sarcoidosis were older at the age of symptom onset, more likely to have comorbidities, and more likely to develop heart failure symptoms over time. From an ECG perspective, PR prolongation and high-grade atrioventricular (AV) block were exclusively associated with cardiac sar-

TABLE 8.1   Differential diagnosis of right-dominant arrhythmogenic cardiomyopathy, aka ARVC

Right-dominant ACM	
Idiopathic VT	Arising from the RVOT
	Arising from other sites in the heart
Cardiac sarcoidosis	.
Structural diseases of the heart	Atrial septal defect
	Abnormal pulmonary venous return
	Ebstein's anomaly
	Congenital pulmonary regurgitation
	Pulmonary artery hypertension
	Pectus excavatum
	Congenital absence of left pericardium
Athlete's heart	
Myocarditis	

coidosis. One of the variables that can distinguish these 2 conditions is the presence of first-degree or higher degrees of AV block, including complete AV block, which are only seen in patients with cardiac sarcoidosis. I have never seen an ARVC patient with first-degree or higher levels of AV block. **Table 8.2** highlights some of the clinical variables that are of value in distinguishing ARVC from cardiac sarcoidosis and idiopathic VT. From an MRI perspective, significant LV dysfunction, myocardial delayed enhancement of the septum, and mediastinal lymphadenopathy were more often seen in those with cardiac sarcoidosis. It is also important not to misdiagnose idiopathic VT as ARVC. We have found that the results of signal-averaged electrocardiogram (SAECG) are often misleading, and we do not rely on this diagnostic test. Similar, epsilon waves have been shown to be of little diagnostic value for ARVC.[7] Finally, the Bordeaux group have reported that a high-dose isoproterenol infusion (45 mcg/min for 3 minutes) can help identify true ARVC.[8] Patients with ARVC will demonstrate frequent multimorphic runs of VT. The response to programmed electrical stimulation and catheter ablation is also of value.

A final diagnosis to be considered in a patient with possible ARVC is myocarditis. It is now well recognized that patients with ARVC can present with chest pain, troponin leaks, and ECG changes. This type of presentation is most common with mutations in desmoplakin and is usually associated with LV involvement.[9,10]

Differential Diagnosis of Left-Dominant and Biventricular ALVC

Although ARVD/C is predominantly a disease of the RV,[11,12] it is now well established that involvement of the LV may occur, particularly when MRI is used to detect subtle abnormalities in LV function and also in patients with advanced disease. Left-dominant arrhythmogenic cardiomyopathy also is defined by early disease of the LV, often affecting the posterolateral LV wall, in the absence of significant RV systolic dysfunction. Left-dominant disease is more commonly seen in patients with desmoplakin or phospholamban (*PLN*) mutations.[13–15] Bhonsale et al. reported the genotype–phenotype relationships in 577 patients and family members with desmosomal or nondesmosomal mutation. LV dysfunction was seen in 78 (14%) of the patients. Twenty-eight (5%) experienced heart failure during follow-up. *PKP-2* carriers were least likely to have LV dysfunction, whereas those with a *DSP* mutation were more likely to have LV dysfunction. Patients with multiple mutations had a more than 3-fold increased risk of LV dysfunction and heart failure.

The differential diagnosis of left-dominant and biventricular ALVC is shown in **Table 8.3**. As noted above, the differential diagnosis includes cardiac sarcoidosis[6] and myocarditis.[9,10] Other conditions that need to be considered include dilated cardiomyopathy, Chagas disease, neuromuscular cardiomyopathy, and athlete's heart.

TABLE 8.2 Distinguishing features of ARVC versus idiopathic RVOT tachycardia versus cardiac sarcoidosis

	ARVC	IDIOPATHIC RVOT VT	CARDIAC SARCOIDOSIS
Familial	Yes	No	No
Genetic testing	Positive (60%)	Negative	Negative
Endurance exercise	Almost always present	No impact	No impact
Age	13–45	Any age	> 40 years
Gender	50/50	50/50	50/50
Symptoms	Asymptomatic or palpitations, syncope, sudden death	Asymptomatic, palpitations, syncope	Asymptomatic or palpitations, syncope, sudden death, CHF
Presenting arrhythmia	Premature ventricular complexes (PVCs), nonsustained ventricular tachycardia (NSVT), sustained VT, ventricular fibrillation (VF)	PVCs, NSVT, sustained VT	PVCs, NSVT, sustained VT, VF
VT morphology	Left bundle superior axis most typical but any morphology	Left bundle inferior axis	Right bundle branch block (RBBB) consistent with LV origin most common, but may be any morphology
ECG findings	T-wave inversion V_2, V_3, +/– beyond, also inferior leads possible. Terminal activation delay, atypical RBBB	Normal ECG	Highly variable; first- or higher-degree AV block possible
Biopsy	Myocyte loss with fibrofatty replacement	Normal	Noncaseating granulomas
Multiple PVC or VT morphologies	May be present	Not present	May be present
Programmed electrical stimulation	Inducible VT, often with multiple morphologies	One morphology, often with isoproterenol	Single of multiple VT morphologies
Response to high-dose isoproterenol	Runs of multimorphic NSVT or sustained VT	PVC suppression or monomorphic PVCs or VT	Not well described
Response to catheter ablation	VT control with endocardial and/or epicardial substrate ablation	Curative with focal ablation	Low efficacy of VT ablation using substrate ablation
VT mechanism	Reentrant, triggered, and/or automatic	Triggered or automatic	Reentrant
Imaging	Dilated RV with decreased function and regional wall motion abnormalities	Normal	Delayed enhancement of the septum, mediastinal lymphadenopathy

TABLE 8.3   Differential diagnosis of ALVC

Left-dominant arrhythmogenic cardiomyopathy	
Cardiac sarcoidosis	
Structural diseases of the heart	Dilated cardiomyopathy
	Chagas heart disease
	Neuromuscular cardiomyopathies (muscular dystrophies and myofibrillar myopathies)
	Congenital ventricular aneurysms
	Pulmonary artery hypertension
	Pectus excavatum
	Congenital absence of left pericardium
Athlete's heart	
Myocarditis	

The 2019 HRS Expert Consensus Statement on Arrhythmogenic Cardiomyopathy

In 2019 HRS published a consensus document on a new entity: "arrhythmogenic cardiomyopathy." They defined ACM as an "arrhythmogenic disorder of myocardium not secondary to ischemic, hypertensive, or valvular disease. ACM incorporates a broad spectrum of genetic, systemic, infectious, and inflammatory disorders." The document goes on to state, "This designation includes but is not limited to arrhythmogenic right ventricular cardiomyopathy, arrhythmogenic left ventricular cardiomyopathy, ion channel abnormalities, amyloidosis, and left ventricular noncompaction." The recommendation also says that genetic testing is indicated for all patients with ACM and includes recommendations for exercise restriction and implantable cardioverter-defibrillator (ICD) implantation. With respect to diagnosis, the document suggests that if a patient presents with ventricular dysfunction and an arrhythmia, ACM is present. The next step is excluding other systemic disorders like sarcoidosis, myocarditis, Chagas disease, and amyloidosis. The document also describes a spectrum of disease, with right-dominant ACM, formerly called ARVC, occurring due to mutations in desmosomal proteins and left-dominant and biventricular ACM occurring due to mutations in genes that are involved with the cytoskeleton, sarcoplasmic reticulum, ion channel, and mitochondria.

Summary

ARVC is an inherited cardiomyopathy characterized clinically by VAs, sudden death, and structural abnormalities predominantly of the RV. It is now well recognized that ARVC is often a biventricular or left-dominant condition. When this condition presents with a left-dominant phenotype, it is often referred to as ALVC.

The diagnosis of ARVC is challenging and requires a careful clinical history, including family and exercise history, as well a variety of diagnostic tests including an ECG, Holter, cardiac MRI, and genetic testing. In this chapter we have outlined the differential diagnosis for ARVC and ALVC and have also introduced the HRS 2019 consensus document on ACM.

References

1. Marcus FI, Fontaine GH, Guiraudon G, et al. Right ventricular dysplasia: A report of 24 adult cases. *Circulation.* 1982;65(2):384–398.

2. Hamid MS, Norman M, Quraishi A, et al. Prospective evaluation of relatives for familial arrhythmogenic right ventricular cardiomyopathy/dysplasia reveals a need to broaden diagnostic criteria. *J Am Coll Cardiol.* 2002;40(8):1445–1450.

3. Corrado D, van Tintelen PJ, McKenna WJ, et al. Arrhythmogenic right ventricular cardiomyopathy: Evaluation of the current diagnostic criteria and differential diagnosis. *Eur Heart J.* 2020;41(14):1414–1429.

4. Towbin JA, McKenna WJ, Abrams DJ, et al. 2019 HRS expert consensus statement on evaluation, risk stratification, and management of arrhythmogenic cardiomyopathy: Executive summary. *Heart Rhythm.* 2019;16(11):e373–e407.

5. Marcus FI, McKenna WJ, Sherrill D, et al. Diagnosis of arrhythmogenic right ventricular cardiomyopathy/dysplasia: Proposed modification of the Task Force Criteria. *Eur Heart J.* 2010;31(7):806–814.

6. Philips B, Madhavan S, James CA, et al. Arrhythmogenic right ventricular dysplasia/cardiomyopathy and cardiac sarcoidosis: Distinguishing features when the diagnosis is unclear. *Circ Arrhythm Electrophysiol.* 2014 Apr;7(2):230–236.

7. Platonov PG, Calkins H, Hauer RN, et al. High interobserver variability in the assessment of epsilon waves: Implications for diagnosis of arrhythmogenic right ventricular cardiomyopathy/dysplasia. *Heart Rhythm.* 2016;13(1):208–216.

8. Denis A, Sacher F, Derval N, et al. Diagnostic value of isoproterenol testing in arrhythmogenic right ventricular cardiomyopathy. *Circ Arrhythm Electrophysiol.* 2014;7(4):590–597.

9. Protonotarios A, Wicks E, Ashworth M, et al. Prevalence of ^{18}F-fluorodeoxyglucose positron emission tomography abnormalities in patients with arrhythmogenic right ventricular cardiomyopathy. *Int J Cardiol.* 2019;284:99–104.

10. Lopez-Ayala JM, Pastor-Quirante F, Gonzalez-Carrillo J, et al. Genetics of myocarditis in arrhythmogenic right ventricular dysplasia. *Heart Rhythm.* 2015;12(4):766–773.

11. Corrado D, Basso C, Judge DP. Arrhythmogenic cardiomyopathy. *Circ Res.* 2017;121(7):784–802.

12. Groeneweg JA, Bhonsale A, James CA, et al. Clinical presentation, long-term follow-up, and outcomes of 1001 arrhythmogenic right ventricular dysplasia/cardiomyopathy patients and family members. *Circ Cardiovasc Genet.* 2015;8(3):437–446.

13. Bhonsale A, Groeneweg JA, James CA, et al. Impact of genotype on clinical course in arrhythmogenic right ventricular dysplasia/cardiomyopathy-associated mutation carriers. *Eur Heart J.* 2015;36(14):847–855.

14. Sen-Chowdhry S, Syrris P, Ward D, Asimaki A, Sevdalis E, McKenna WJ. Clinical and genetic characterization of families with arrhythmogenic right ventricular dysplasia/cardiomyopathy provides novel insights into patterns of disease expression. *Circulation.* 2007;115:1710–1720.

15. Sen-Chowdhry S, Syrris P, Prasad SK, et al. Left-dominant arrhythmogenic cardiomyopathy: An under-recognized clinical entity. *J Am Coll Cardiol.* 2008;52(25):2175–2187.

16. Berte B, Denis A, Amraoui S, et al. Characterization of the left-sided substrate in arrhythmogenic right ventricular cardiomyopathy. *Circ Arrhythm Electrophysiol.* 2015;8(6):1403–1412.

9

Life-Threatening Arrhythmias Without Overt Clinical Disease: "Concealed" Arrhythmogenic Right Ventricular Cardiomyopathy

Christopher Semsarian, MBBS, PhD, MPH;
Jodie Ingles, GradDipGenCouns, PhD, MPH

Introduction

Arrhythmogenic right ventricular cardiomyopathy (ARVC) is an inherited myocardial disorder characterized by loss of cardiomyocytes and their replacement with fibrofatty tissue. Although the right ventricle (RV) is predominantly affected, the left ventricle (LV) is also commonly involved.[1] The clinical prevalence of ARVC is highly variable in different countries, with estimates of up to 1 in 2000 people. Our understanding of ARVC continues to evolve in parallel with wider recognition of the condition, more comprehensive phenotype investigation and characterization, and deeper understanding of the underlying genetic mechanisms.[2,3] With better imaging modalities and the increasing utility and availability of genetic testing, ARVC is beginning to be recognized and diagnosed earlier in life.

Clinical Phases of ARVC

The clinical phases of ARVC are summarized in **Figure 9.1**. ARVC commonly presents with symptomatic RV arrhythmias, often accompanied by overt RV structural changes such as dilatation and dyskinesis. The diseases can progress to gradual loss of RV myocardium, global RV dysfunction, and clinical evidence of RV failure. In the later clinical phases of ARVC, there can be significant LV involvement, leading to biventricular heart failure and death.[1] These overt clinical phases are not always sequential in their development and progression. Each of the clinical phases is relatively easy to identify through standard cardiac investigations, such as echocardiogram, Holter monitoring, electrocardiography (ECG), and cardiac magnetic resonance imaging (MRI), in association with interpretation and assessment by clinicians with expertise in cardiomyopathies.

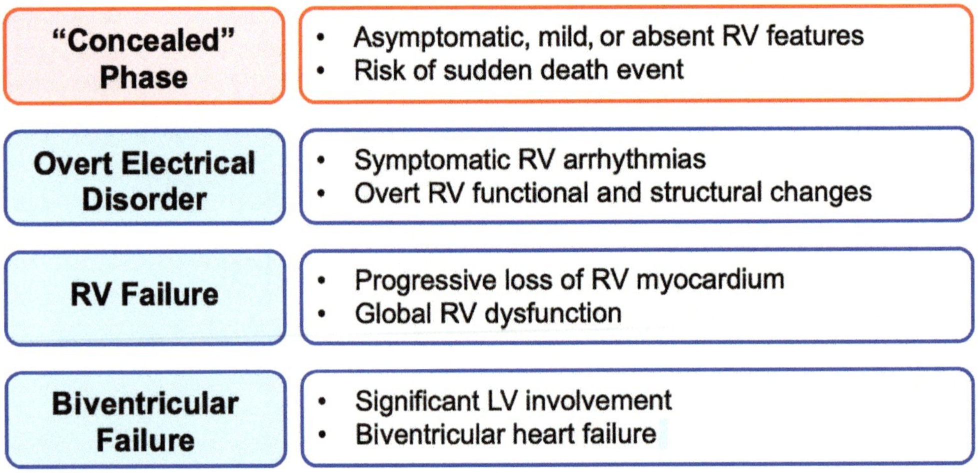

"Concealed" Phase	• Asymptomatic, mild, or absent RV features • Risk of sudden death event
Overt Electrical Disorder	• Symptomatic RV arrhythmias • Overt RV functional and structural changes
RV Failure	• Progressive loss of RV myocardium • Global RV dysfunction
Biventricular Failure	• Significant LV involvement • Biventricular heart failure

FIGURE 9.1 Clinical phases of ARVC.

Concealed Phase of ARVC

In recent years, there has been an increasing awareness of a potentially earlier "preclinical" or "concealed" phase of ARVC.[4] The word "concealed" in the Oxford English Dictionary is defined as *to be kept hidden or secret, or out of sight*. This describes the concealed phase of ARVC precisely.

This new phase of disease is intricately linked to the progress in defining the genetic causes of ARVC and the redefining of ARVC as a disease of the desmosome and intercalated disc. There are 5 main desmosomal genes associated with ARVC: plakophilin-2 (*PKP2*), desmoplakin (*DSP*), desmoglein (*DSG2*), desmocollin (*DSC2*), and plakoglobin (*JUP*). The increasing use of clinical genetic testing in ARVC has fostered the development of a new cohort of individuals at risk of developing ARVC, but with no overt clinical or structural signs of disease, so-called gene mutation carriers or genotype-positive, phenotype-negative individuals. These individuals are asymptomatic, have mild or absent RV features, and represent a concealed phase of ARVC with no clear understanding about how these individuals should be managed, how frequently they should be monitored, what their risk of sud-den death is, and whether any prevention strategies should be initiated.

Of all the disease genes known in ARVC, plakophilin-2 (*PKP2*) is the most commonly implicated, and an integral component of the desmosome, with important roles in cell–cell adhesion. Pathogenic variants in *PKP2* are a well-established cause of ARVC, and life-threatening arrhythmias have generally been shown only to occur in mutation carriers with clear structural disease on imaging.[5] *PKP2* is important for transcription of genes that control intracellular calcium cycling, and it is hypothesized this newly described disease mechanism could lead to life-threatening arrhythmias in humans in the absence of structural disease.[6] Despite this, the arrhyth-mic risk is not seen prior to development of an overt phenotype.[7,8]

Representative Cases of Concealed ARVC

To illustrate the potential concealed phase of ARVC, 4 unrelated probands are described here who presented due to an unexplained sudden cardiac arrest with overt structurally normal hearts in early adulthood, with caus-ative loss of function variants in the *PKP2* gene subsequently identified.[4] The genetic findings in these 4 probands are summarized (see **Table 9.1**), while a brief clinical description for each proband is summarized here.

Proband 1

Patient AWF1 presented at age 29 years after suffering a resuscitated cardiac arrest during her first pregnancy, while playing netball, a high-exertion sport popular in Commonwealth countries. She underwent implantable cardioverter-defibrillator (ICD) placement, and cardiac investigations failed to reveal a cardiac diagnosis. A 12-lead ECG showed a QTc of 435 ms and no other abnormalities noted (**Figure 9.2**, Panel A). Transthoracic echocardiography revealed no overt structural disease with normal LV and RV size and function. Genetic testing identified a pathogenic splice variant c.2489+1G>A in *PKP2*, previously reported in

at least 25 ARVC cases. Family screening was unremarkable; however, a great-grandmother died suddenly, aged 29 years, with "fibrofatty degeneration of the heart and cardiac dilatation" noted on the death certificate in 1925. Over a follow-up period of 7 years, AFW1 has since had multiple appropriate therapies for rapid ventricular arrhythmias (VAs) from her ICD and has developed structural and functional RV changes.

Proband 2

Patient BTT1 presented at age 23 years after a resuscitated cardiac arrest while playing football and suffered significant neurological impairment. There was no prior medical history and no significant family history. Comprehensive cardiac investigations revealed no overt abnormalities. Genetic testing identified a pathogenic duplication resulting in

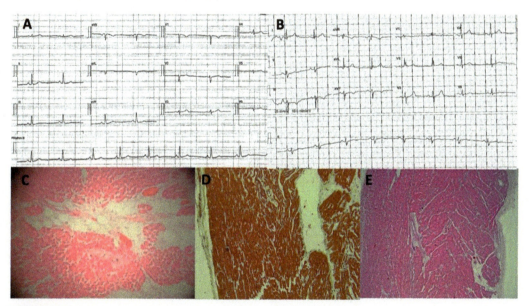

FIGURE 9.2 Clinical and pathological features in concealed phase ARVC cases.
Panel A: The 12-lead ECG for AWF1 prearrest shows normal sinus rhythm. **Panel B:** A premorbid 12-lead electrocardiogram for QW1 shows normal sinus rhythm, right bundle branch block (RBBB) pattern, and inferior T-wave inversion. **Panel C:** QW1 postmortem section of RV 4× objective hematoxylin and eosin stain (site not determined) shows some fibrosis and fat infiltration, considered abnormal but nondiagnostic of ARVC. **Panels D** and **E:** AYD1 postmortem section of RV outflow tract (RVOT) shows normal morphology, without fibrosis, inflammation, or excessive fat infiltration; respectively, (**D**) 4× objective Movat's pentachrome stain and (**E**) 2× objective hematoxylin and eosin stain.

a frameshift and premature stop codon in *PKP2*, c.2361dupT; p.Leu788Serfs*3. The variant has not been previously reported and is absent from control populations. One year following the cardiac arrest, BTT1 had > 900 ventricular ectopic beats documented on 24-hour Holter monitoring, consistent with a diagnosis of ARVC.

Proband 3

Patient QW1 suffered a sudden cardiac death (SCD) at age 30 years while in bed. He had reported presyncope on exertion in the days preceding his death. A premorbid ECG 12 months prior to the death showed sinus rhythm (Figure 9.2, Panel B). Postmortem examination revealed mild LV dilation (40 mm). The heart weight was 710 grams, which within the context of a body mass index of 36.2 kg/m^2 was considered normal. Sections of RV, LV, and septum showed some areas of fat infiltration and fibrosis of the myocardium, suggestive but not diagnostic of ARVC (Figure 9.2, Panel C). Research-based exome sequencing identified a pathogenic nonsense variant, c.2391C>A; p.Tyr797Ter in *PKP2*, which was shown to not be present in both parents, that is, the pathogenic *PKP2* variant in the deceased occurred as a *de novo* event.

Proband 4

Patient AYD1 suffered an SCD at age 15 years following a minor physical altercation. The family history was unremarkable. Postmortem examination was performed by an experienced forensic pathologist and showed no abnormalities. Minimal fatty streaking of the aorta was reported, and heart weight was within normal limits. Sections of RVOT showed normal morphology, and no fibrosis, inflammation, or excessive fat infiltration was evident (Figure 9.2, Panels D and E). Postmortem genetic testing was performed as part of a national prospective study[9] and a 2 base-pair deletion in *PKP2* resulting in a frameshift and stop codon was identified: c.252_255ddelTGAG; p.Glu85Metfs*26.

In summary, these 4 young individuals presented with sudden cardiac arrest events with structurally normal hearts and causative loss-of-function *PKP2* variants (Table 9.1). Two died, while two survived the sudden cardiac arrest. The genetic findings and young presentation are key features, and contrary to previous studies suggesting nonsense variants are associated with later-onset disease.[10] All 4 individuals were probands, that is, the first to present clinically in their respective families, and not individuals detected by cascade family screening. In our experience in Sydney, Australia, these concealed ARVC cases presenting with an SCD event accounted for 4 out of 173 (2%) unexplained SCD events.[4] While arrhythmic risk is not generally reported prior to structural disease, most knowledge about *PKP2* carriers comes from observational studies of ARVC cohorts. Recently, reports from colleagues in Canada suggest this concealed phase of ARVC is not limited to *PKP2* carriers, but also presents in carriers of pathogenic variants in the *DSP* gene.[11–13] Importantly, these ARVC gene carriers who present in a concealed phase of disease do not fulfill 2010 ARVC Task Force Criteria (TFC)[14] despite their significant risk of life-threatening VAs and sudden death.

TABLE 9.1 Genetic findings in concealed ARVC sudden death event cases

PROBAND	*PKP2* VARIANT DETAILS	ACMG/AMP VARIANT CLASSIFICATION
AWF1	c.2489+1 G>A (splice variant)	Pathogenic
BTT1	p.Leu744Serfs*3	Likely pathogenic
QW1	p.Tyr797Ter	Pathogenic
AYD1	p.Glu85Metfs*26	Likely pathogenic

Abbreviations: fs, frameshift; Ter, termination; ACMG/AMP, American College of Medical Genetics and Genomics and Association of Medical Pathologists.

Molecular Insights of Concealed ARVC and Sudden Death

Why an ARVC gene carrier with no overt structural disease can present with a sudden cardiac event remains unclear. However, one possibility is that the genetic changes found in disease genes such as *PKP2* or *DSP* may trigger key molecular and cellular events leading to a predisposition to the development of VAs in the absence of major or minor diagnostic criteria for ARVC. An elegant study recently published by the group led by Drs. Mario Delmar and Marina Cerrone[15] provides fascinating insights into the potential mechanisms and substrates that may explain the arrhythmic predisposition in the concealed phase of ARVC. Using multiple imaging, biochemical, and mass spectrometry approaches in cardiomyocyte (CM) specific, tamoxifen-activated, *PKP2* knockout mice, the authors demonstrate multiple molecular perturbations, including Ca^{2+} dysregulation mediated by both RyR2 phosphorylation and connexin43 membrane potential changes.[15] The findings support the notion that *PKP2* loss-of-function variants trigger molecular changes that precede the development of structural cardiomyopathy changes, and explain the observation of a concealed phase of disease in ARVC patients (Figure 9.3).

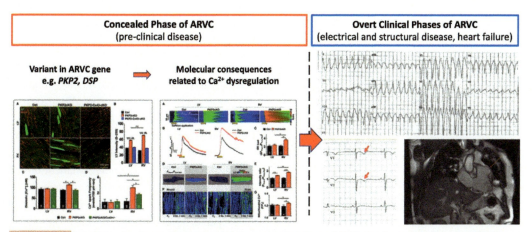

FIGURE 9.3 Potential molecular mechanisms underlying concealed phase of ARVC. A pathogenic variant in an ARVC gene triggers subclinical molecular changes including Ca^{2+} dysregulation, leading to an arrhythmogenic substrate *prior to* development of overt clinical ARVC, with structural changes and arrhythmias. (Figure reproduced from Kim et al., *Circulation.* 2019;140:1015–1030.[15])

Clinical Implications of "Concealed Phase" ARVC

The emergence of the concealed phase of ARVC has important implications and presents a clinical conundrum in terms of management of asymptomatic ARVC gene carriers who do not have overt structural disease, and do not fulfill the 2010 ARVC Task Force Criteria (TFC). The overwhelming clinical issue is, therefore, how do we investigate and manage asymptomatic patients who carry likely pathogenic or pathogenic genetic variants, such as in *PKP2* or *DSP*, but have no overt signs of structural abnormalities? Most cardiologists will primarily rely on the 12-lead ECG, echocardiography, and cardiac MRI to assess any structural or electrical evidence of ARVC. In a gene carrier where there is no evidence of structural disease on comprehensive imaging, how would such a patient be assessed for risk of arrhythmias and sudden death? Is a normal ECG, an exercise test, and 24-hour ambulatory ECG monitoring a sufficient level of investigation to reassure the patient that his or her risk of a life-threatening arrhythmia and sudden death is low? Should further arrhythmic risk be assessed by additional investigations such as electrophysiological testing, or testing for potential new biomarkers[16] with enhanced sensitivity for earlier disease risk detection? If all these investigations are normal, how often should the patient be reviewed?

An additional important unanswered clinical question relates to whether the risk of an arrhythmic event prior to structural disease is also applicable to at-risk relatives shown to be gene positive for the family variant detected via cascade family screening, or whether the concealed phase of ARVC is only confined to probands, as in the four cases described. Amongst ARVC families, probands are in many cases the most severely affected, suggesting a complex underlying disease etiology, with emerging evidence pointing to a role for additional nongenetic and environmental factors, such as high-level exercise, altering the natural history of ARVC.[17] This element of unpredictability creates a clinical dilemma in sudden death risk stratification and overwhelmingly highlights a limitation of the 2010 ARVC TFC and an area requiring further collaborative global research.

Take-Home Messages

The concealed phase of ARVC is a relatively new clinical phenomenon with many unanswered questions, presenting significant diagnostic and management challenges to the treating clinician. In summary:

- The **concealed phase in ARVC** is an important stage in the disease.
- Individuals (the probands) in this phase are **at risk of SCD events** and may be difficult to identify.
- Genotype status, especially **loss-of-function *PKP2* variants**, may be an important marker, along with variants in other ARVC genes such as *DSP*.
- These findings have important implications for **risk stratification** in ARVC.

References

1. Towbin JA, McKenna WJ, Abrams DJ, et al. 2019 HRS expert consensus statement on evaluation, risk stratification, and management of arrhythmogenic cardiomyopathy. *Heart Rhythm.* 2019;16:e301–e372.
2. Hamilton-Craig C, McGavigan A, Semsarian C, et al. The Cardiac Society of Australia and New Zealand Position Statement on the diagnosis and management of arrhythmogenic right ventricular cardiomyopathy (2019 Update). *Heart Lung Circ.* 2020;29:40–48.
3. Oomen A, Semsarian C, Puranik R, Sy RW. Diagnosis of arrhythmogenic right ventricular cardiomyopathy: Progress and pitfalls. *Heart Lung Circ.* 2018;27:1310–1317.

4. Ingles J, Bagnall RD, Yeates L, et al. Concealed arrhythmogenic right ventricular cardiomyopathy in sudden unexplained cardiac death events. *Circ Genom Precis Med.* 2018;11:e002355.

5. te Riele AS, Bhonsale A, James CA, et al. Incremental value of cardiac magnetic resonance imaging in arrhythmic risk stratification of arrhythmogenic right ventricular dysplasia/cardiomyopathy-associated desmosomal mutation carriers. *J Am Coll Cardiol.* 2013;62:1761–1769.

6. Cerrone M, Montnach J, Lin X, et al. Plakophilin-2 is required for transcription of genes that control calcium cycling and cardiac rhythm. *Nat Commun.* 2017;8:106.

7. te Riele AS, James CA, Groeneweg JA, et al. Approach to family screening in arrhythmogenic right ventricular dysplasia/cardiomyopathy. *Eur Heart J.* 2016;37:755–763.

8. Dalal D, James C, Devanagondi R, et al. Penetrance of mutations in plakophilin-2 among families with arrhythmogenic right ventricular dysplasia/cardiomyopathy. *J Am Coll Cardiol.* 2006;48:1416–1424.

9. Bagnall RD, Weintraub RG, Ingles J, et al. A prospective study of sudden cardiac death among children and young adults. *N Engl J Med.* 2016;374:2441–2452.

10. Alcalde M, Campuzano O, Berne P, et al. Stop-gain mutations in PKP2 are associated with a later age of onset of arrhythmogenic right ventricular cardiomyopathy. *PLoS One.* 2014;9:e100560.

11. Cheung CC, Davies B, Krahn AD. Letter by Cheung et al regarding article, "Concealed arrhythmogenic right ventricular cardiomyopathy in sudden unexplained cardiac death events". *Circ Genom Precis Med.* 2019;12:e002447.

12. Krahn AD, Healey JS, Chauhan V, et al. Systematic assessment of patients with unexplained cardiac arrest: Cardiac Arrest Survivors With Preserved Ejection Fraction Registry (CASPER). *Circulation.* 2009;120:278–285.

13. Mellor G, Laksman ZWM, Tadros R, et al. Genetic testing in the evaluation of unexplained cardiac arrest: From the CASPER (Cardiac Arrest Survivors With Preserved Ejection Fraction Registry). *Circ Cardiovasc Genet.* 2017;10.

14. Marcus FI, McKenna WJ, Sherrill D, et al. Diagnosis of arrhythmogenic right ventricular cardiomyopathy/dysplasia: Proposed modification of the Task Force Criteria. *Circulation.* 2010;121:1533–1541.

15. Kim JC, Perez-Hernandez M, Alvarado FJ, et al. Disruption of Ca(2+)i homeostasis and connexin 43 hemichannel function in the right ventricle precedes overt arrhythmogenic cardiomyopathy in plakophilin-2-deficient mice. *Circulation.* 2019;140:1015–1030.

16. Chatterjee D, Fatah M, Akdis D, et al. An autoantibody identifies arrhythmogenic right ventricular cardiomyopathy and participates in its pathogenesis. *Eur Heart J.* 2018;39:3932–3944.

17. James CA, Bhonsale A, Tichnell C, et al. Exercise increases age-related penetrance and arrhythmic risk in arrhythmogenic right ventricular dysplasia/cardiomyopathy-associated desmosomal mutation carriers. *J Am Coll Cardiol.* 2013;62:1290–1297.

10

Genotype-Phenotype Correlations in ACM: The Chinese Experience

Liang Chen, MD, PhD; Jiangping Song, MD, PhD

Introduction

Arrhythmogenic cardiomyopathy (ACM) is an inherited primary cardiomyopathy[1,2] that is one of the leading causes of sudden cardiac death (SCD) in young people (35 years) in western countries. Genetic analyses have revealed that ~50% of ACM cases carry desmosomal gene mutations, including *PKP2*, *JUP*, *DSP*, *DSG2*, and *DSC2*.[3] Nondesmosomal genes have also been implicated in ACM patients, such as *TMEM43*, *DES*, *LMNA*, *TTN*, *LMNA*, *PLN*, *CTNNA3*, *CDH2*, and *FLNC*. Genotype–phenotype correlation studies among transatlantic cohorts have shown that discrete clinical features and outcomes occur in patients with different mutations.[4] Most previous ACM studies have examined Caucasian patients, whereas few studies have included patients from East Asia.[5] Recently, next-generation sequencing (NGS) has allowed studies to include the con-current sequencing of all of the ACM-related genes for entire patient cohorts.

Genotype-Clinical Phenotype in Fuwai ACM Cohort

As the largest cardiovascular specialty hospital in China with more than 1400 patient beds, Fuwai Hospital, also known as the National Center for Cardiovascular Diseases, has established the largest ACM cohort in China. Patients from this cohort are mostly of Han Chinese descent and come from multiple areas all over China. Using NGS, including whole-exome sequencing (WES) and gene panels containing more than 60 cardiomyopathy-related genes, we illuminated the genetic background of part of ACM patients. We further characterize the genetic and clinical features of Chinese ACM patients, to explore potential correlations and to characterize the inheritance of ACM in term of specific gene mutations among this

East Asian population. We also illuminated the genotype and pathological characteristics of end-stage ACM hearts from 60 heart transplantation (HTx) patients.

The sequenced ACM patients by NGS consisted of 118 unrelated individuals (81 males), of which 106 patients fulfilled the modified diagnostic 2010 Task Force Criteria (TFC) for ACM, 7 patients were classified as borderline ACM, and 5 patients were classified as possible cases. Sixty pathogenic mutations were detected in 67 patients, of whom 7 individuals (6%) carried digenic mutations (**Figure 10.1**). Different from Caucasian populations, the Chinese ACM cohort contained more *DSG2* mutation carriers. We detected 12 *DSG2* mutations in 20 probands (17%), including 9 homozygous missense mutations, 6 compound mutations, 3 heterozygous mutations, and 2 digenic mutations. It is noteworthy that 17 out of 20 ACM patients with *DSG2* carried double (multiple) mutations in the Chinese ACM cohort. We detected 19 *PKP2* mutations in 22 probands (19%), among whom 16 patients carried a single

heterozygous mutation, 2 carried compound mutations, and 4 had digenic mutations. Interestingly, the founder mutation in Netherlands *PLN* p.Arg14del is also identified in 4 Han Chinese patients with ACM.[6]

Analysis of PKP2 Mutation Carriers

As *PKP2* is the most prevalent mutant gene causing ACM in East Asia as well as western countries, in another study we focused on the *PKP2* patients with single or multiple mutations.[7] Based on DNA sequencing, we identified 22 patients with *PKP2* mutation among 118 individuals. Further, we applied RNA sequencing of 27 explanted heart tissues to improve the genetic diagnosis as described by Cummings et al.[8] for the purpose of detecting cryptic splicing events. Interestingly, by adapting the integrative analysis of RNA sequencing and DNA sequencing, we identified 2 aberrant splicing mutations in one patient who was defined as nonmutation by DNA sequencing. Moreover, we confirmed genomic variants of *PKP2* in the vicinity of

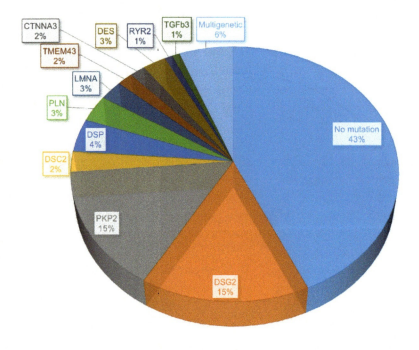

FIGURE 10.1 The distribution of gene mutations among 118 ACM patients is presented.

aberrant splicing, and 2 rare intronic variants were identified: The variant c.224-3T>C led to exon2 skipping, and the variant c.2490-6T>C led to exon13 extension. Our RNA sequencing data confirmed the pathogenesis of these intronic variants. Thus, we obtained 5 ACM patients with compound mutations of *PKP2*, called recessive *PKP2*. Recessive *PKP2* variant positive probands had typical ACM characteristics with left ventricular (LV) involvement, and none of them had extracardiac lesions. All patients with recessive *PKP2* variants had early onset of ACM prior to 18 years (from 2 years up to 18 years of age). Signs and symptoms related to heart failure were detected in 4 patients (80%), and all patients had a left ventricular ejection fraction (LVEF) < 50%. Two patients underwent HTx due to end-stage heart failure, and 2 died from heart failure during follow-up.

We compared the clinical characteristics of patients with recessive *PKP2* variants (n = 5) to patients with a single heterozygous variant in *PKP2* (n = 17). Patients with recessive *PKP2* variants showed significantly more prevalent early onset of ACM-related symptoms (11.8 ± 5.9 years vs. 27.4 ± 8.4 years, *P* < 0.001), with a higher rate of abdominal distension (40% vs. 0%, *P* = 0.040) and bilateral edema (60% vs. 0%, *P* = 0.006), but a lower rate of palpitations (0% vs. 100%, *P* < 0.001). Moreover, patients with recessive *PKP2* variants had more severe impaired LV structure and function, with a higher rate of LV dilation (40% vs. 0%, *P* = 0.060) and dyskinesia (100% vs. 0%, *P* < 0.001), and a lower LVEF (27.4 ± 9.8% vs. 61.9 ± 6.0%, *P* < 0.001). Patients with *PKP2* recessive variants had both worse HTx/death-free and major adverse cardiac event (MACE)-free survival rates as compared to patients with a single *PKP2* heterozygous variant (*P* < 0.001 and *P* = 0.003, respectively) (**Figure 10.2**). By using combined implementation of WGS RNAseq, this study demonstrates that recessive variants in *PKP2* may

contribute to early-onset ACM with severe heart failure. These findings may play a role in risk stratification of ACM based on genetic testing in clinical practice.

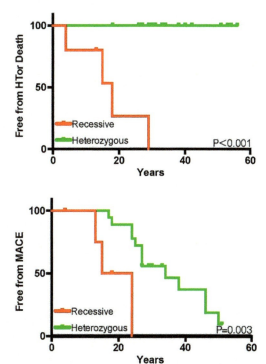

FIGURE 10.2   Kaplan–Meier analyses. **Top Panel:** Cumulative freedom from MACE and HTx/death (**Bottom Panel**) presents in patients with *PKP2* recessive variants and those with *PKP2* heterozygous variants.

Analysis of DSG2 Mutation Carriers

As another star gene in the Fuwai ACM cohort, *DSG2* mutations are carried in 17% of patients, most of which were even compound or homozygous mutations, including one impressive variant *DSG2* c.1592T>G. We then focused on 8 ACM patients with homozygous *DSG2* c.1592T>G mutations.[9] Age of initial ACM-related symptoms ranged from 14 to 34 years old (mean age 24.5 ± 5.9). Five probands started with palpitation, syncope, and ventricular arrhythmias (VAs); one patient was found to have an electrocardiogram (ECG) abnormality as well as right ventricle (RV) enlargement and dysfunction without apparent symptoms; one patient presented with VAs and RV dominant cardiac dysfunction during the perinatal period, and received a HTx as a result of progressive biventricular heart failure; and the youngest proband had a fulminant heart failure course, requiring HTx within 6 months after the first symptoms. The pathological presentation by cardiac magnetic resonance (CMR) imaging included extensive delayed enhancement and fibrofatty tissue replacement with significant dilation in the RV. Interventricular septum showed delayed enhancement at the distal level adjacent to the cardiac apex under the 4-chamber section. Additionally, the LV was affected as reflected by cardiac dysfunction (LVEF < 50%) and fibrofatty infiltration (shown by late gadolinium enhancement [LGE]) mainly at the posterolateral free wall. Therefore, it was noteworthy that DSG2 c.1592T>G patients were prone to LV dysfunction, which increased the risk for HTx and premature death.

Clinical and genetic evaluations were also performed among relatives of 7 probands. One patient refused family screening in this study. Among 31 relatives, 23 were identified to be genotype positive, including 1 homozygous variant and 22 heterozygous variant carriers. In addition to 1 family member with a homozygous variant who was diagnosed with ACM and received implantable cardioverter-defibrillator (ICD) implantation in our hospital. Six of 22 heterozygous family members showed mild ACM-related symptoms, including 2 with palpitations; 2 received radiofrequency catheter ablation due to VAs, one with T-wave inversion and one with mild RV dilation. No heterozygous variant carriers fulfilled the definite diagnosis criteria, and none of them have received therapy by the present time. Penetrance analysis proved that all (100%) of the homozygotes were diagnosed with ACM; 25% of heterozygous variant car-

riers presented moderate ACM symptoms at senior age, and no ACM-related symptoms were discovered in family members without mutation.

Population Prevelance of ACM Genotypes

We further reviewed and found 4 previous reports about this variant from Japan, Chinese Taiwan, and South and East China, all from East Asia, but none in other regions (**Figure 10.3**). To investigate whether probands carrying the DSG2 c.1592T>G have a common ancestor, we performed haplotype analysis using 4 polymorphic microsatellites (D18S847, D18S963, D18S36, D18S47) and 5 SNPs in vicinity to DSG2 c.1592T>G locus. A shared haplotype, spanning N450 kb, was identified in both alleles of 8 probands carrying homozygous c.1592T>G and one allele of 4 index patients with heterozygous c.1592T>G variant, indicating that these families most likely had a common founder (Figure 10.3). Meanwhile, we also screened these markers among 23 family members with c.1592T>G variant and demonstrated that all mutation carriers share the same haplotype within the allele of c.1592T>G variant. Interestingly, we also screened the DSG2 c.1592T>G variant among 400 non-ARVC cardiomyopathies in our cardiac center, and only 2 patients (0.25%) carried a heterozygous variant, which is a similar allele frequency in the East Asia population. This suggested that DSG2 c.1592T>G carriers mainly exhibit the phenotype of ACM without overlap with other cardiomyopathies.

This work identified for the first time a homozygous founder variant (c.1592T>G) of DSG2 in East Asia, which was highly prevalent among Chinese ACM patients with full penetrance for homozygous carriers; this result suggested an urgent demand for genetic counseling for the index patients and their relatives carrying the heterozygous variant.[9] In

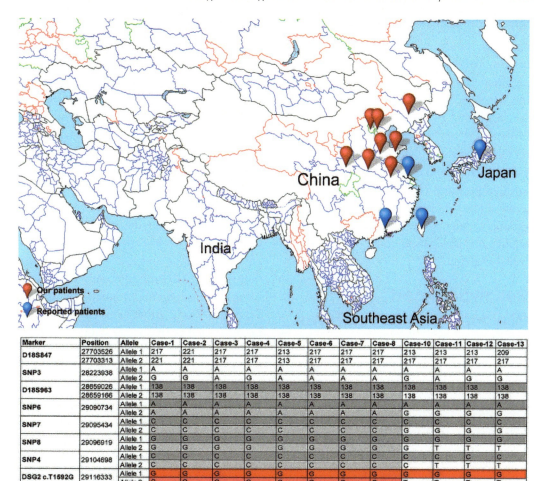

Marker	Position	Allele	Case-1	Case-2	Case-3	Case-4	Case-5	Case-6	Case-7	Case-8	Case-10	Case-11	Case-12	Case-13
D18S847	27703526	Allele 1	217	221	217	217	213	217	217	217	213	213	213	209
	27703313	Allele 2	221	221	217	217	213	217	217	217	217	217	217	217
SNP3	28223938	Allele 1	A	A	A	A	A	A	A	A	A	A	A	A
		Allele 2	G	G	A	G	A	A	A	A	G	A	G	G
D18S963	28659026	Allele 1	138	138	138	138	138	138	138	138	138	138	138	138
	28659166	Allele 2	138	138	138	138	138	138	138	138	138	138	138	138
SNP6	29090734	Allele 1	A	A	A	A	A	A	A	A	A	A	A	A
		Allele 2	A	A	A	A	A	A	A	A	G	G	G	G
SNP7	29095434	Allele 1	C	C	C	C	C	C	C	C	C	C	C	C
		Allele 2	C	C	C	C	C	C	C	C	G	G	G	G
SNP8	29096919	Allele 1	G	G	G	G	G	G	G	G	G	G	G	G
		Allele 2	G	G	G	G	G	G	G	G	G	T	T	T
SNP4	29104698	Allele 1	C	C	C	C	C	C	C	C	C	C	C	C
		Allele 2	C	C	C	C	C	C	C	C	C	T	T	T
DSG2 c.T1592G	29116333	Allele 1	G	G	G	G	G	G	G	G	G	G	G	G
		Allele 2	G	G	G	G	G	G	G	G	T	T	T	T
D18S36	29164196	Allele 1	139	139	139	139	139	139	139	139	139	139	139	139
	29164339	Allele 2	139	143	139	139	141	139	139	139	152	139	145	137
D18S47	29781230	Allele 1	201	197	197	197	197	197	201	197	197	201	197	197
	29781429	Allele 2	201	201	203	197	197	197	201	197	197	211	203	205

FIGURE 10.3 Genetic epidemiology of *DSG2* c.1592T>G variant. Distribution of the families carrying *DSG2* c.1592T>G variant in East Asia (**top**). The **red balloons** represent Fuwai cohort patients, and **blue** balloons are those previously reported by others. Genetic analysis revealed 8 homozygous mutation probands shared a haplotype spanning N450 kb (**bottom**). Case means the homozygous c.1592T>G probands, and Con means the ACM patients without this variant.

summary, this study extended our knowledge regarding the genetic heterogeneity of ACM in East Asia and highlighted the regional importance of certain gene mutations. Defining selection criteria by which rare variants are considered causal is mandatory; indeed, this study demonstrated that stringent criteria should be established, taking into account cohort location and ethnicity in order to avoid misinterpretation of genetic variants. Systemic studies of disease prevalence and gene-variants frequency are required to determine population divergences underlying phenotypic variability.[10]

Genotype-Based Clinicopathology: The Fuwai Classification of ACM

Another important genotype–phenotype study from the China Fuwai ACM cohort is the novel genotype-based clinicopathology classification of end-stage ACM based on explanted hearts.[11] ACM is an inherited cardiomyopathy characterized by the fibrofatty replacement of the myocardium predominantly in the RV.[1,12] It was first systematically described and demonstrated to be an essential cause of SCD among young adults in the 1980s.[13,14] A series of subsequent studies were reported to clarify the clinicopathology in order to distinguish it from myocarditis and adipos, cordis.[15–19] LV involvement verified by autopsy expanded the spectrum of manifestations beyond an isolated RV disease.[20] Afterward, the left-dominant subtype was also identified, which supported the adoption of a broader term "arrhythmogenic cardiomyopathy" (ACM).[21] As the signature character of ACM hearts, the distribution and extent of fibrofatty replacement of the myocardium are known to be heterogeneous between individuals. Pathologists have been trying to categorize ACM since the 1990s.[17,18,22] However, early pathological examinations were limited

due to disease diagnosis based on the original TFC, and the genetic information was not available at that time. Based on 60 ACM explanted hearts with standard pathology examinations obtained from Fuwai Hospital from 2005 to 2018, we established a digital pathology and image segmentation platform to meticulously analyze the fatty, fibrotic, and myocardial tissue distribution in 6 representative transmural specimens (4 in the LV and 2 in the RV) at midventricular level for each heart. By analyzing the circumferential as well as epicardial-to-endocardial distribution of fibrofatty tissue, we were able to distinguish 4 distinct ACM clusters for end-stage disease using an unsupervised consensus clustering algorithm. Each of these clusters appeared to be associated with specific clinical features and genetic findings.

Transplanted ACM hearts in Cluster 1 exhibited transmural fatty replacement of the entire RV and in the posterolateral wall of the LV. Most of these patients had early-onset disease and mainly carried desmosomal mutations with the exception of *DSP*. They experienced ventricular tachyarrhythmias and received an ICD more commonly. In addition, they underwent heart transplantation (HTx) at younger age. The patients in this cluster represented end-stage disease of classical desmosomal ARVC. In the validation cohort, the disease showed a consistent progressive pattern, starting from regional involvement in the RV, gradually spreading to the entire RV, and later involving the LV. On surface ECG, precordial QRS voltage decreased continuously during the course of disease. Cluster 2 ACM hearts were affected by fibrofatty infiltration mainly in the anterior wall of the RV. There was only a little fat and limited interstitial fibrosis in the LV. Nevertheless, fibrosis was extending to the full thickness of the LV, resulting in lower LVEF compared with that observed in Cluster 1. The patients were mostly carriers of nondesmosomal gene mutations, such as *LMNA*, *DES*, and *PLN*. Cluster 3 ACM hearts showed moderate fibrofatty infiltration of the RV, whereas fibrofatty replacement of the LV was more severe as compared with the previous 2 subtypes. Thus, Cluster 3 is associated with biventricular disease. All *DSP* mutation carriers were in this group. Cluster 4 cases showed typical LV-dominant ACM with minimal or no RV involvement, and none of these patients had a known genetic mutation

(**Figure 10.4**). In a further step, we validated their results in a cohort of 92 ACM patients by analyzing late-gadolinium.

This work was named the "Fuwai Classification" by ACM experts Profs. Firat Duru and Richard N. W. Hauer once published.[23] The implications of the Fuwai Classification of ACM are also manifold. Patients with desmosomal mutations, with the exception of *DSP*, presented classic pathological remodeling

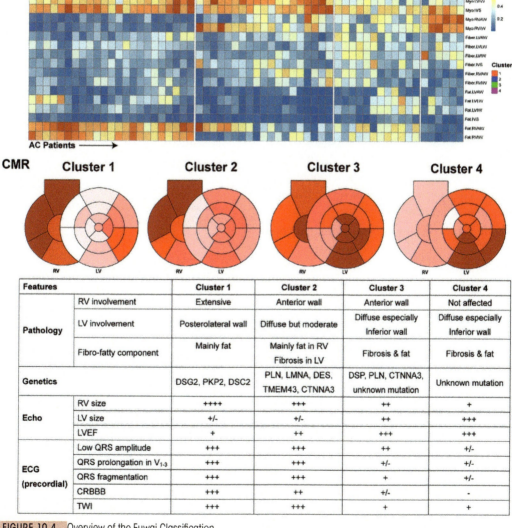

Features		Cluster 1	Cluster 2	Cluster 3	Cluster 4
Pathology	RV involvement	Extensive	Anterior wall	Anterior wall	Not affected
	LV involvement	Posterolateral wall	Diffuse but moderate	Diffuse especially Inferior wall	Diffuse especially Inferior wall
	Fibro-fatty component	Mainly fat	Mainly fat in RV Fibrosis in LV	Fibrosis & fat	Fibrosis & fat
Genetics		DSG2, PKP2, DSC2	PLN, LMNA, DES, TMEM43, CTNNA3	DSP, PLN, CTNNA3, unknown mutation	Unknown mutation
Echo	RV size	++++	+++	++	+
	LV size	+/-	+/-	++	+++
	LVEF	+	++	+++	+++
ECG (precordial)	Low QRS amplitude	+++	+++	++	+/-
	QRS prolongation in V_{1-3}	+++	+++	+/-	+/-
	QRS fragmentation	+++	+++	+	+/-
	CRBBB	+++	++	+/-	-
	TWI	+++	+++	+	+

FIGURE 10.4 Overview of the Fuwai Classification.

defined as Cluster 1 with extensive fat replacement in the entire RV and fibrofatty infiltration in the posterolateral wall of the LV. This subtype could be defined as "desmosomal cardiomyopathy" or classical ARVC as previously suggested.[24] Similar to previous reports,[1,21] *DSP* mutation carriers presented with serious LV involvement (Cluster 3), suggesting different pathogenesis from other desmosome gene carriers. And thus, it remains uncertain to include *DSP* mutation carrier in the classical "desmosomal cardiomyopathy." Nondesmosomal gene carriers such as *LMNA* and *DES* were mainly affected by fibrofatty replacement at the regional area of the RV and limited fibrosis infiltration of the LV, which were categorized as Cluster 2. *PLN* 14del was demonstrated to be associated with ACM and dilated cardiomyopathy (DCM) with serious LV involvement.[25] Our 5 *PLN* 14del carriers were distributed in both Cluster 2 (4 cases) and Cluster 3. These distinct pathology characteristics of different genotypes indicate different pathogenic mechanisms among these subtypes. Additionally, there are some patients with the left-dominant ACM phenotype who have no underlying mutation (Cluster 4).

In summary, this study sheds light on our knowledge on phenotype–histopathology–genotype correlations for ACM and provides a novel classification with 4 distinctly different clusters in describing this unique, multifaceted disease. This work was also awarded with the best clinical research prize at the Zurich International Symposium on Arrhythmogenic Cardiomyopathy, which was voted by a 7-member Prize Selection Committee from transatlantic centers.

Conclusion

The ACM group at Fuwai Hospital in Beijing, China, has primarily illuminated the genetic background of Chinese ACM patients and established the correlation between genotype and clinical phenotype as well as genotype and histopathology characteristics. These findings make contributions to the diagnosis, risk stratification, family screening, and potential mechanisms studies in Chinese ACM patients. Our multidisciplinary team at Fuwai Hospital is investigating the multiple facets of ACM from clinicopathology, electrophysiology, genotype, and molecular phenotype approaches to mechanism and rescue studies. This group is also open for any potential collaboration to study the comparison of the patient populations from Asia and the Caucasus, to study the effect of exercise in eastern and western countries, and to study the pathogenesis and therapeutic strategies to this disease.

References

1. Corrado D, Link MS, Calkins H. Arrhythmogenic right ventricular cardiomyopathy. *N Engl J Med.* 2017;376(1):61–72.

2. Gandjbakhch E, Redheuil A, Pousset F, Charron P, Frank R. Clinical diagnosis, imaging, and genetics of arrhythmogenic right ventricular cardiomyopathy/dysplasia: JACC State-of-the-Art Review. *J Am Coll Cardiol.* 2018;72(7):784–804.

3. Corrado D, Basso C, Judge DP. Arrhythmogenic cardiomyopathy. *Circ Res.* 2017;121(7): 784–802.

4. Bhonsale A, Groeneweg JA, James CA, et al. Impact of genotype on clinical course in arrhythmogenic right ventricular dysplasia/cardiomyopathy-associated mutation carriers. *Eur Heart J.* 2015;36(14):847–855.

5. Bao J, Wang J, Yao Y, et al. Correlation of ventricular arrhythmias with genotype in arrhythmogenic right ventricular cardiomyopathy. *Circ Cardiovasc Genet.* 2013;6(6):552–526.

6. van der Zwaag PA, van Rijsingen IA, de Ruiter R, et al. Recurrent and founder mutations in the Netherlands-Phospholamban p.Arg14del mutation causes arrhythmogenic cardiomyopathy. *Neth Heart J.* 2013;21(6):286–293.

7. Chen K, Rao M, Guo G, et al. Recessive variants in plakophilin-2 contributes to early-onset arrhythmogenic cardiomyopathy with severe heart failure. *Europace.* 2019;21(6):970–977.

8. Cummings BB, Marshall JL, Tukiainen T, et al. Improving genetic diagnosis in Mendelian disease with transcriptome sequencing. *Sci Transl Med.* 2017;9:386.

9. Chen L, Rao M, Chen X, et al. A founder homozygous DSG2 variant in East Asia results in ARVC with full penetrance and heart failure phenotype. *Int J Cardiol.* 2019;274:263–270.

10. Celeghin R, Pilichou K. The complex molecular genetics of arrhythmogenic cardiomyopathy. *Int J Cardiol.* 2019;284:59–60.

11. Chen L, Song J, Chen X, et al. A novel genotype-based clinicopathology classification of arrhythmogenic cardiomyopathy provides novel insights into disease progression. *Eur Heart J.* 2019;40(21):1690–1703.

12. Basso C, Corrado D, Marcus FI, Nava A, Thiene G. Arrhythmogenic right ventricular cardiomyopathy. *Lancet.* 2009;373(9671):1289–1300.

13. Thiene G, Nava A, Corrado D, Rossi L, Pennelli N. Right ventricular cardiomyopathy and sudden death in young people. *N Engl J Med.* 1988;318(3):129–133.

14. Marcus FI, Fontaine GH, Guiraudon G, et al. Right ventricular dysplasia: A report of 24 adult cases. *Circulation.* 1982;65(2):384–398.

15. Thiene G, Corrado D, Nava A, et al. Right ventricular cardiomyopathy: Is there evidence of an inflammatory aetiology? *Eur Heart J.* 1991;12 Suppl D: 22–25.

16. Hofmann R, Trappe HJ, Klein H, Kemnitz J. Chronic (or healed) myocarditis mimicking arrhythmogenic right ventricular dysplasia. *Eur Heart J.* 1993;14(5):717–720.

17. Basso C, Thiene G, Corrado D, Angelini A, Nava A, Valente M. Arrhythmogenic right ventricular cardiomyopathy: Dysplasia, dystrophy, or myocarditis? *Circulation.* 1996;94(5):983–991.

18. Burke AP, Farb A, Tashko G, Virmani R. Arrhythmogenic right ventricular cardiomyopathy and fatty replacement of the right ventricular myocardium: Are they different diseases? *Circulation.* 1998;97(16):1571–1580.

19. Basso C, Thiene G. Adipositas cordis, fatty infiltration of the right ventricle, and arrhythmogenic right ventricular cardiomyopathy: Just a matter of fat? *Cardiovasc Pathol.* 2005;14(1):37–41.

20. Sen-Chowdhry S, Syrris P, Ward D, Asimaki A, Sevdalis E, McKenna WJ. Clinical and genetic characterization of families with arrhythmogenic right ventricular dysplasia/cardiomyopathy provides novel insights into patterns of disease expression. *Circulation.* 2007;115(13):1710–1720.

21. Sen-Chowdhry S, Syrris P, Prasad SK, et al. Left-dominant arrhythmogenic cardiomyopathy: An under-recognized clinical entity. *J Am Coll Cardiol.* 2008;52(25):2175–1287.

22. Corrado D, Basso C, Thiene G, et al. Spectrum of clinicopathologic manifestations of arrhythmogenic right ventricular cardiomyopathy/dysplasia: A multicenter study. *J Am Coll Cardiol.* 1997;30(6):1512–1520.

23. Duru F, Hauer RNW. Multiple facets of arrhythmogenic cardiomyopathy: The Fuwai classification of a unique disease based on clinical features, histopathology, and genotype. *Eur Heart J.* 2019;40(21):1704–1746.

24. Thiene G. The research venture in arrhythmogenic right ventricular cardiomyopathy: A paradigm of translational medicine. *Eur Heart J.* 2015;36(14):837–846.

25. te Rijdt WP, van Tintelen JP, Vink A, et al. Phospholamban p.Arg14del cardiomyopathy is characterized by phospholamban aggregates, aggresomes, and autophagic degradation. *Histopathology.* 2016;69(4):542–550.

11

Biomarkers in Inherited Arrhythmias: Arrhythmogenic Right Ventricular Cardiomyopathy and Beyond

Robert M. Hamilton, MD, MHSc

Introduction

Laboratory-based biomarkers (biological markers) are substances that can be measured accurately and reproducibly in the body or its products and predict the incidence or outcome of disease, including effects of treatments or interventions.[1] For inherited arrhythmia disorders, some biomarkers may provide the potential for disease diagnosis despite a varying range of genetic or pathophysiological etiologies, whether known or unknown.[2,3] Some biomarkers may also provide a measure of risk between different individuals with the same disease mutation. Thus, biomarkers can often be used to both augment and complement genetic diagnostics.

Biomarkers can be classified into several types: diagnostic, predictive, companion, or prognostic. A diagnostic biomarker typically allows detection of disease in a minimally invasive way. The term *predictive* can have two meanings. For the purpose of this article, *predictive* means that a biomarker can identify patients who will develop disease, prior to exhibiting clinical features that are diagnostic of that disease. The term *predictive* is also used to indicate that a biomarker can identify which patient may respond to a therapy. For this article, we will use the term *companion* for biomarkers that are used to guide therapy. Such companion biomarkers may identify candidate patients for a therapy, and may also be used to guide the response to that therapy. Finally, prognostic biomarkers are those that effectively contribute to the risk stratification of a patient, such as the risk of major arrhythmic events in inherited arrhythmia conditions.

Disease biomarkers may take many forms, but two common forms of biomarkers include serum or plasma proteins, and more recently circulating ribonucleic acids. A challenge of assessing protein biomarkers is their diversity and extreme range of concentrations within circulating serum or plasma. Evolving mass spectrometry methods have improved the ability to detect very small quantities of biomarker proteins, but highly abundant proteins tend to obscure the detection of potential low-concentration biomarkers. The most common strategy to resolve this problem is depletion of high-abundance proteins, but this process needs to be standardized, and the depletion process may alter the prtein biomarker of interest.

Pathogenic disease processes are usually responsible for the generation of circulating protein biomarkers. However, these circulating protein biomarkers are likely to be recognized as foreign in the circulation, and multiple pathways may lead to degradation of the potential biomarker signal. Proteins that are pathologically released to the circulation and expose an immunologically unrecognized peptide sequence (cryptic epitope) to the immune system may provide a method to amplify rather than degrade a biomarker signal. The immune system can generate a response to this cryptic epitope, creating a robust autoantibody response. Thus, by measuring the presence of antibodies to the pathologically released protein, rather than the protein itself, a strong biomarker signal may be identified. We have taken advantage

of this phenomenon to identify biomarkers for arrhythmogenic right ventricular cardiomyopathy (ARVC, see **Figure 11.1**)[3] and Brugada syndrome (BrS),[2] as described below. Additionally, this autoimmune response may occasionally contribute to disease pathogenesis as well.

Novel Biomarker for Arrhythmogenic Right Ventricular Cardiomyopathy (ARVC)

We noted that rare patients with apparent ARVC could be identified who had no family history of disease and no identifiable disease mutation. We also noted that desmosomal disorders are represented in skin, and that a specific group of skin diseases, pemphigus, are associated with autoantibodies to skin desmosomal proteins desmoglein-1 and desmoglein-3. We therefore hypothesized that ARVC might occasionally be associated with autoantibodies to components of the cardiac desmosome. Since antibodies are traditionally considered to bind extracellular targets, we chose to focus on the cadherins of the cardiac desmosome that project an extracellular motif: desmocollin-2 (DSC2) and desmoglein-2 (DSG2). Also, as cardiac intercalated disk junctions may

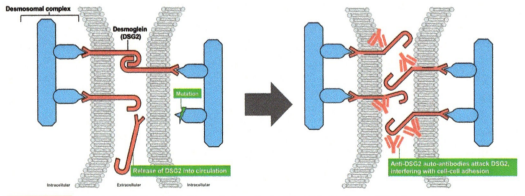

FIGURE 11.1 **Left Panel:** Mutations within the cardiomyocyte desmosomal complex result in release of DSG2 into the circulation, stimulating an autoimmune response. **Right Panel:** Anti-DSG2 antibodies result in distortion of DSG2 and failure to crosslink. (Reproduced from Chatterjee et al., *Eur Heart J*. 2018;39(44):3932–3944.[3])

incorporate more complex junctions (area composita) that include components of adherens junctions and its N-cadherin (NCAD) protein that is also implicated as a genetic cause of ARVC, we also assessed this molecule.

We purchased commercial human DSC2, DSG2, and NCAD proteins, ran them on western blots to confirm their identity, and used this western blot platform to detect their respective autoantibodies in ARVC patient sera. In our discovery cohorts, 12 of 12 sera from subjects with definite ARVC and 7 of 8 sera from subjects with borderline ARVC had anti-DSG2 antibodies, whereas among 12 commercial control sera, we identified only faint staining in one (this was later identified to be against a different portion of the DSG2 protein than that typically targeted in ARVC patient sera). Anti-DSG2 antibodies were also present in 25 of 25 sera from a separate validation cohort of definite ARVC subjects from the Zurich ARVC program, and absent in a second set of controls from a different commercial source. Interestingly, antibodies to human DSG2 protein were also identified in 10 of 10 ARVC-affected Boxer dogs compared to 18 healthy dogs (16 Boxers, 2 other breeds) with no pedigree history of ARVC (human and canine DSG2 protein are 77% homologous). The autoantibody assay was also developed into an enzyme-linked immunosorbent assay that demonstrated excellent discrimination of ARVC patients from controls.[3]

Despite the strong performance of our developed assay, it is challenging to translate the original assay to one that can be performed routinely in a clinical laboratory setting (whether hospital-based or through a healthcare diagnostics company). The difficulty is that the whole DSG2 protein is insoluble and requires an Fc tag to make it soluble. An Fc tag is the constant region of immunoglobulin heavy-chain, and it is often used to solubilize as well as purify proteins, but it is immunoreactive in and of itself. Therefore, the immuno-

reactivity of this tag must be "blocked" before the remaining portion of the molecule can be used to assay for anti-DSG2 antibodies. These blocking steps are well described in our original publication (and the supplementary material online),[3] but remain a challenge for routine use in a clinical laboratory. Therefore, we have switched to an assay that utilizes only the two oligopeptide epitope regions that are targeted by antibodies from ARVC patients: the extracellular cadherin 4 (EC4) and extracellular cadherin 5/extracellular articulating (EC5/EA) regions. These oligopeptides are soluble and can be generated reproducibly and in high purity at low cost, making then ideal for a simple clinical laboratory assay.

Novel Biomarker Profile for Brugada Syndrome

We had noted increasing evidence in the literature identifying inflammation in BrS[4,5] and recognized that although they are usually unique phenotypes (and genotypes where known), there is occasionally overlap between ARVC and BrS. We hypothesized that autoimmunity might be present in BrS and potentially contribute to the recognized inflammation, but we did not have a specific indication as to what the target proteins of those autoantibodies might be. We therefore developed an antibody discovery platform by generating a 2D gel of myocardial proteins from a normal heart, separated by molecular weight and isoelectric pH, exposing them to sera from BrS patients and normal controls, and identifying any targets of identified autoantibodies by mass spectrometry. Using this platform, we identified a unique profile of autoantibodies to actins (α-cardiac and α-skeletal muscle), keratin (we identified keratin-24), and connexin43 in sera from every subject in discovery (n = 3) and validation (n = 18) cohorts who met the most recent consensus conference definition of probable or definite BrS (Shanghai score

≥ 3.5), which was absent in sera from 32 control individuals.[2] A biomarker for BrS is an important advance, as a disease-causing gene (SCN5A or other) is only identified in 25% to 30% of cases, and the clinical diagnosis has been dependent on a type 1 Brugada pattern electrocardiogram (ECG), which is a fluctuant finding, and frequently requires a modified lead ECG and/or provocation with a sodium channel-blocking drug.

The reason for antibodies to actins, keratin, and connexin43 was unclear, and we therefore sought to assess the expression of these proteins in myocardium from BrS subjects (in heart tissue from one decedent and endomyocardial biopsies from 9 patients). Actin protein staining switched from a fine filamentous pattern to rope-like bundles of protein. Connexin43 showed somewhat larger aggregates within cells. Keratin demonstrated large aggregates of protein rather than the nor-

mal fine, speckled pattern. We also assessed the expression of the cardiac sodium channel protein Na$_v$1.5, which also demonstrated large aggregates in myocardium from BrS subjects.[2]

If protein misexpression also occurs in cell or zebrafish embryo models of BrS, it may provide a useful signal for the assessment of high-throughput screening of potentially therapeutic small molecules. We speculate that these misexpressed proteins within the cytoplasm may undergo disposal from the cell, exposing cryptic epitopes that trigger an autoimmune response (**Figure 11.2**). Regardless of etiology, the presence of misexpressed proteins in the myocardium of BrS subjects suggests that this assessment could assist in the postmortem diagnosis of BrS as the etiology of sudden cardiac death (SCD).

Our ARVC enzyme-linked immunosorbent assay (ELISA) identifies disease, distinguishes it from other cardiomyopathies, and

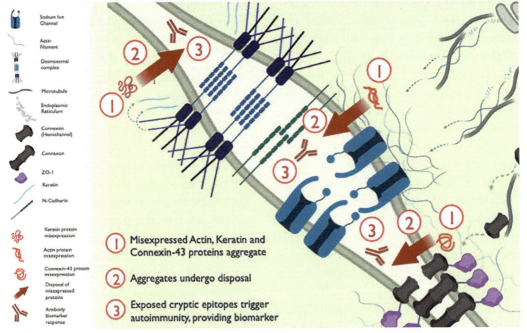

FIGURE 11.2 (**1**) As part of the pathophysiology of BrS, actin, keratin, and connexin43 proteins are misexpressed and form aggregates within cardiomyocytes. (**2**) These protein aggregates undergo cell disposal. (**3**) As a result, cryptic epitopes of these proteins are exposed to the immune system, resulting in the generation of specific autoantibodies, creating a biomarker profile for the disease. (Reproduced from Chatterjee et al., *Eur Heart J.* 2020;41:2878–2890.[2])

tracks with the ARVC Task Force category of disease (**Figure 11.3**, left panel). Our BrS ELISA can effectively distinguish BrS from ARVC and other cardiomyopathies (Figure 11.3, right panel).

Other Biomarkers in Inherited Arrhythmias

Several other proteins can act as biomarkers within ARVC, particularly to identify specific subgroups. Cardiac ankyrin repeat protein,[6] pro-atrial natriuretic peptide, and heat shock protein 70[7] are increased in myocardium from ARVC patients with heart failure, with the latter demonstrating increased serum levels as well.[7] Mean plasma bridging integrator 1 levels are decreased in patients with ARVC and heart failure.[8] Plasma N-terminal pro-brain natriuretic peptide (Nt-BNP) level is significantly higher in patients with right ventricular (RV) dysfunction than in patients without.[9] Plasma levels of soluble ST2, an interleukin 1 receptor molecule, is higher in patients with ventricular arrhythmias (VAs) than in patients without,[10] although we have not seen this rela-

tionship in young patients (< 18 years old, unpublished findings). Elevated serum testosterone levels in males and decreased estradiol levels in females are independently associated with major adverse cardiac events in ARVC,[11] and the effect of testosterone in males was confirmed in an independent study.[12] Plasma levels of certain microRNAs can also predict VAs in ARVC.[13]

Serum biomarkers have been assessed in hypertrophic cardiomyopathy (HCM) more than any other arrhythmia condition. As early as 1992, Maisch identified antimyolemmal antibodies in 78%, and antifibril antibodies in 43%, of sera from patients with HCM.[14] Plasma Nt-BNP levels correlate with LV end-diastolic septal thickness and mass index and are negatively correlated with left ventricular (LV) diastolic internal dimension.[15] HCM patients with both high cardiac troponin I and Nt-BNP values had an 11.7-fold increased risk of cardiovascular events compared with those with low values.[16] Elevated high-sensitivity cardiac troponin T is also an independent predictor of cardiovascular events,[17] and is a marker of ongoing myocardial fibrosis.[18]

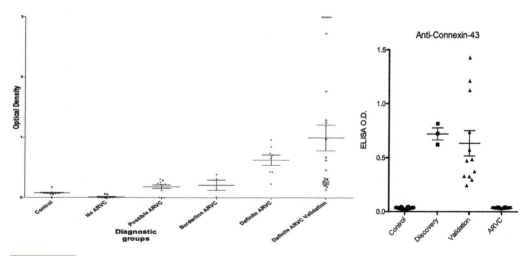

FIGURE 11.3   **Left Panel:** Anti-DSG2 antibody optical density increases from control or "No ARVC" patients to "Possible," "Borderline," and "Definite" categories. **Right Panel:** Anti-connexin43 (and other BrS autoantibodies) separate BrS subjects from ARVC subjects.

Low levels of apelin, a natural antagonist of angiotensin II, are also associated with myocardial fibrosis in HCM.[19] Higher levels of soluble ST2 (previously mentioned) are seen in HCM patients with nonsustained ventricular tachycardia (VT),[20] and galectin-3 levels are predictive of SCD in HCM.[21] Recently, a multiplex biomarker panel of six proteins (aldolase fructose-bisphosphate A, complement C3, glutathione S-transferase omega 1, Ras suppressor protein 1, talin 1, and thrombospondin 1) was found to identify HCM and correlate with phenotype severity.[22] A study of cardiac biomarkers in pediatric cardiomyopathy is ongoing.[23]

Autoimmunity as a Target for Therapy in Inherited Arrhythmias (ACM)

We identified that the level of anti-DSG2 antibody has a moderately large, positive, linear association with premature ventricular complex (PVC) burden in ARVC patients (R^2 = 0.49).[3] Using a robotic system we developed to measure dye transfer through gap junctions in normal induced pluripotent stem cell-derived cardiac myocytes (iPSC-CMs),[24–26] exposure to IgG from the serum of ARVC subjects (as well as commercial anti-DSG2 antibodies) demonstrated a 20% reduction in linear dye transfer between cells (36% reduction in area of cells), indicating that anti-DSG2 antibodies reduce gap junction function, a feature common to all forms of ARVC to date. We have now extended these studies to other platforms that measure CM function and conduction,[27] including the Xcelligence RTCA Cardio platform, a novel label-free platform that can measure CM conduction (CardioPyrate), and 3D constructs of iPSC-CMs.

Autoimmunity may represent a therapeutic target in ARVC. Traditional "anti-immune" therapies include prednisone, dexamethasone, methotrexate, cyclophosphamide, combinations of these drugs, or drugs such as nonsteroidal anti-inflammatory drugs (NSAIDs) or disease-modifying antirheumatic drugs (DMARDs, e.g., Plaquenil). Increasingly more targeted anti-immune therapies are being developed, such as anti-TNF agents, monoclonal antibodies, modulators of the immune system (e.g., FcRn receptor antagonists), and cell-based treatments. Essentially, none of these have yet been evaluated in ARVC. We have used pulsed steroid therapy in a few patients where cardiac inflammation was first confirmed by positron emission tomography (PET) with 2-deoxy-2-[fluorine[18]] fluoro-D-glucose (^{18}F-FDG PET), with transient suppression of arrhythmic storm (unpublished data). We are currently evaluating the development of synthetic Bi-specific T cell engaging antibodies to potentially treat ACM by engaging the patient's natural killer T cells to target the B cell/plasma cell clones responsible for anti-DSG2 antibody production (under a University of Toronto Medicine by Design grant). Under this grant, we have also proposed to develop chimeric autoantibody receptor (CAAR) T cells to perform this function, similar to the use of CAAR T cells to treat pemphigus by targeting anti-DSG3 producing cells (an endeavor that recently received two rounds of major investment; Cabaletta Bio). It will become increasingly important to assess new therapies in appropriate experimental models that include assessment of autoimmune components of the disease and their response to therapy.

References

1. Strimbu K, Tavel JA. What are biomarkers? *Curr Opin HIV AIDS.* 2010;5(6):463–466.
2. Chatterjee D, Pieroni M, Fatah M, et al. An autoantibody profile detects Brugada syndrome and identifies abnormally expressed myocardial proteins. *Eur Heart J.* 2020;41:2878–2890.

3. Chatterjee D, Fatah M, Akdis D, et al. An autoantibody identifies arrhythmogenic right ventricular cardiomyopathy and participates in its pathogenesis. *Eur Heart J.* 2018;39(44):3932–3944.

4. Pieroni M, Notarstefano P, Oliva A, et al. Electroanatomic and pathologic right ventricular outflow tract abnormalities in patients with Brugada syndrome. *J Am Coll Cardiol.* 2018;72(22):2747–2757.

5. Li A, Tung R, Shivkumar K, Bradfield JS. Brugada syndrome-malignant phenotype associated with acute cardiac inflammation? *Heart Rhythm Case Rep.* 2017;3(8):384–388.

6. Wei YJ, Cui CJ, Huang YX, Zhang XL, Zhang H, Hu SS. Upregulated expression of cardiac ankyrin repeat protein in human failing hearts due to arrhythmogenic right ventricular cardiomyopathy. *Eur J Heart Fail.* 2009;11(6):559–566.

7. Wei YJ, Huang YX, Shen Y, Cui CJ, Zhang XL, Zhang H, Hu SS. Proteomic analysis reveals significant elevation of heat shock protein 70 in patients with chronic heart failure due to arrhythmogenic right ventricular cardiomyopathy. *Mol Cell Biochem.* 2009;332(1-2):103–111.

8. Hong TT, Cogswell R, James CA, et al. Plasma BIN1 correlates with heart failure and predicts arrhythmia in patients with arrhythmogenic right ventricular cardiomyopathy. *Heart Rhythm.* 2012;9(6):961–967.

9. Cheng H, Lu M, Hou C, et al. Relation between N-terminal pro-brain natriuretic peptide and cardiac remodeling and function assessed by cardiovascular magnetic resonance imaging in patients with arrhythmogenic right ventricular cardiomyopathy. *Am J Cardiol.* 2015;115(3):341–347.

10. Broch K, Leren IS, Saberniak J, Ueland T, Edvardsen T, Gullestad L, Haugaa KH. Soluble ST2 is associated with disease severity in arrhythmogenic right ventricular cardiomyopathy. *Biomarkers.* 2017;22(3-4):367–371.

11. Akdis D, Saguner AM, Shah K, et al. Sex hormones affect outcome in arrhythmogenic right ventricular cardiomyopathy/dysplasia: From a stem cell derived cardiomyocyte-based model to clinical biomarkers of disease outcome. *Eur Heart J.* 2017;38(19):1498–1508.

12. Ren J, Chen L, Zhang N, et al. Plasma testosterone and arrhythmic events in male patients with arrhythmogenic right ventricular cardiomyopathy. *ESC Heart Fail.* 2020;7(4):1547–1559.

13. Yamada S, Hsiao YW, Chang SL, et al. Circulating microRNAs in arrhythmogenic right ventricular cardiomyopathy with ventricular arrhythmia. *Europace.* 2018;20(FI1):f37–f45.

14. Maisch B. Anticardiac antibodies in hypertrophic cardiomyopathy as a marker of severity. *Postgrad Med J.* 1992;68 Suppl 1:S29–S35.

15. Kim SW, Park SW, Lim SH, et al. Amount of left ventricular hypertrophy determines the plasma N-terminal pro-brain natriuretic peptide level in patients with hypertrophic cardiomyopathy and normal left ventricular ejection fraction. *Clin Cardiol.* 2006;29(4):155–160.

16. Kubo T, Kitaoka H, Okawa M, et al. Combined measurements of cardiac troponin I and brain natriuretic peptide are useful for predicting adverse outcomes in hypertrophic cardiomyopathy. *Circ J.* 2011;75(4):919–926.

17. Kubo T, Kitaoka H, Yamanaka S, et al. Significance of high-sensitivity cardiac troponin T in hypertrophic cardiomyopathy. *J Am Coll Cardiol.* 2013;62(14):1252–1259.

18. Kawasaki T, Sakai C, Harimoto K, Yamano M, Miki S, Kamitani T. Usefulness of high-sensitivity cardiac troponin T and brain natriuretic peptide as biomarkers of myocardial fibrosis in patients with hypertrophic cardiomyopathy. *Am J Cardiol.* 2013;112(6):867–872.

19. Zhou Y, Yuan J, Wang Y, Qiao S. Predictive values of apelin for myocardial fibrosis in hypertrophic cardiomyopathy. *Int Heart J.* 2019;60(3):648–655.

20. Gawor M, Spiewak M, Kubik A, Wrobel A, Lutynska A, Marczak M, Grzybowski J. Circulating biomarkers of hypertrophy and fibrosis in patients with hypertrophic cardiomyopathy assessed by cardiac magnetic resonance. *Biomarkers.* 2018;23(7):676–682.

21. Emet S, Dadashov M, Sonsoz MR, et al. Galectin-3: A novel biomarker predicts sud-

den cardiac death in hypertrophic cardiomyopathy. *Am J Med Sci*. 2018;356(6):537–543.

22. Captur G, Heywood WE, Coats C, et al. Identification of a multiplex biomarker panel for hypertrophic cardiomyopathy using quantitative proteomics and machine learning. *Mol Cell Proteomics*. 2020;19(1):114–127.

23. Everitt MD, Wilkinson JD, Shi L, et al. Cardiac biomarkers in pediatric cardiomyopathy: Study design and recruitment results from the pediatric cardiomyopathy registry. *Prog Pediatr Cardiol*. 2019;53:1–10.

24. Fridman MD, Liu J, Sun Y, Hamilton RM. Microinjection technique for assessment of gap junction function. *Methods Mol Biol*. 2016;1437:145–154.

25. Liu J, Siragam V, Chen J, Fridman MD, Hamilton RM, Sun Y. High-throughput measurement of gap junctional intercellular communication. *Am J Physiol Heart Circ Physiol*. 2014;306(12):H1708–H1713.

26. Liu J, Siragam V, Gong Z, et al. Robotic adherent cell injection for characterizing cell-cell communication. *IEEE Trans Biomed Eng*. 2015;62(1):119–125.

27. Wang L, Dou W, Malhi M, et al. Microdevice platform for continuous measurement of contractility, beating rate, and beating rhythm of human-induced pluripotent stem cell-cardiomyocytes inside a controlled incubator environment. *ACS Appl Mater Interfaces*. 2018;10(25):21173–21183.

12

Atrial Fibrillation and ECG Markers of Atrial Involvement in Arrhythmogenic Right Ventricular Cardiomyopathy

Maria A. Baturova, MD, PhD; Pyotr G. Platonov, MD, PhD

Introduction

Arrhythmogenic right ventricular cardiomyopathy (ARVC) is an inherited cardiomyopathy characterized by fibrofatty replacement of the myocardium leading to electric instability[1] and associated with increased risk of cardiac arrhythmias.[1] While studies of arrhythmic substrate in ARVC have understandably been focused on the risk of life-threatening ventricular arrhythmias (VAs), recent studies have drawn attention to atrial fibrillation (AF), which appears to have high prevalence among ARVC patients.[2–4]

Prevalence of Atrial Fibrillation in ARVC

The prevalence of AF ranges from 14% in unselected patients with ascertained ARVC diagnosis,[3] to 24% in ARVC patients with ventricular tachycardias (VTs),[5] up to 42% in ARVC patients who underwent ablation for VAs.[4] The observed difference in the prevalence of atrial arrhythmias between the studies is likely to be due to the patient selection since the highest prevalence was observed among those with VTs representing patients with severe disease phenotype.

Recently, we performed a study with focus on AF prevalence and its association with the severity of the disease in 293 patients with definite ARVC diagnosis and their 141 genotype-positive family members from the Nordic ARVC Registry (www.arvc.dk).[6] The registry was launched in June 2010 and has been recruiting patients previously diagnosed with ARVC using 1994 Task Force Criteria (TFC) and followed in 8 tertiary care centers in Denmark, Norway, or Sweden, covering a population of approximately 14 million.[7,8] The registry has also been prospectively including newly diagnosed patients after 2010 with definite ARVC according to 2010 TFC,[9] and their genotype-positive family members. We have found that AF was observed in 14% of definite ARVC patients at 50 years of age and in only 1 of 141 genotype-positive family members. According to the epidemiological data from the same geographical region, such as the Malmo diet and cancer study,[10] the prevalence of AF for the age group 50 to 55 years is reported to be as low as 1%. Notably, in our study, the prevalence of AF in genotype-positive family members without prominent disease was 0.7%, which is similar to the prevalence in the general population. AF prevalence of 14 times higher than the reported prevalence in the general population of the same age supports the hypothesis that AF might be considered as one of the arrhythmic manifestations of ARVC. The high prevalence of AF in ARVC patients indicates a need for alertness among clinicians to rule out AF and consider primary prevention strategies in regard to thromboembolic complications of AF.

We assessed the association between AF and phenotypical manifestations of ARVC using the diagnostic score[3,11] as a measure of ARVC phenotype severity. The score was calculated as the sum of major and minor criteria in all categories of the 2010 TFC, with each major criterion contributing 2 points and minor criteria contributing 1 point. Starting with the diagnostic score 4, which is a threshold for definite ARVC diagnosis, the prevalence of AF increased along with the increase in the diagnostic score (Somer's d = 0.074, $P < 0.001$, **Figure 12.1**), thus indicating that AF is strongly linked to the disease severity.

Pathophysiologic Mechanisms of AF in ARVC Patients

The mechanisms underlying AF development in ARVC patients are not fully understood. Though we could not exclude the role of pulmonary vein triggers in the development

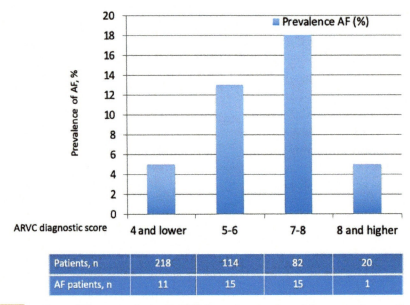

ARVC diagnostic score	4 and lower	5-6	7-8	8 and higher
Patients, n	218	114	82	20
AF patients, n	11	15	15	1

FIGURE 12.1 Prevalence of AF among patients with ARVC diagnosis and carriers of disease-causing genetic variants according to the ARVC diagnostic score based on assignment of 1 point for a minor diagnostic criterion and 2 points for a major diagnostic criterion. The lowest score of 2 corresponds to mutation-carrying status without other disease manifestations (a major diagnostic criterion). (Modified from Baturova et al., *Int J Cardiol.* 2020;298:39–43.[6])

of AF, mechanistically, two principal mechanisms leading to development of AF in ARVC can be considered:

- Hemodynamic consequences of the right ventricular (RV)contractile dysfunction may contribute to right atrial overload, increased stretch, and development of fibrosis in the atrial walls.[12] Left ventricular (LV) involvement in the disease leading to systolic dysfunction may also be associated with complications such as AF and thromboembolic events.[13]

- On the other hand, ARVC has traditionally been considered as a desmosomal disease.[14] Desmosomes are found throughout the cardiac myocardium, including atrial myocardium.[15] Therefore, AF in patients with ARVC may be due to involvement of the atrial myocardium in the disease progression driven by the same desmosomal dysfunction leading to fibrotic transformation as in the ventricles. There are anecdotal reports documenting atrial myocardial involvement in ARVC patients based on postmortem case series[16] and supported by animal studies.[17,18]

P-Wave Indices as Indicators of Atrial Involvement in ARVC

P-wave indices are known electrocardiogram (ECG) markers of atrial abnormalities.[19,20] In earlier studies that addressed atrial remodeling unrelated to ARVC, it has been shown that P-wave duration, P-terminal negative force in lead V_1 (PTF-V_1), P-wave morphology, and P-wave area in lead V_1 reflect electrophysiological and structural abnormalities in the atria.[20,21] It has been shown that P-wave duration is correlated to the extent of atrial fibrosis.[19] Abnormal PTF-V_1 has been shown to be associated with an increase in left atrial volume, and a decrease in left atrial contractile and reservoir function, which represents the filling of the left atrium during ventricular systole.[20]

However, little attention has been paid to P-wave indices in the context of ARVC. Previously, our group addressed this question using P-wave–triggered signal-averaged orthogonal ECG from 40 ARVC patients and compared them with age- and sex-matched healthy control subjects for assessment of P-wave duration and morphology.[22] In addition to a significant P-wave prolongation observed in patients with ARVC, more than one-third of middle-aged ARVC patients presented with atypical P-wave morphology, which was an extremely rare finding in controls.

In order to assess whether abnormalities in P-wave indices represent early or late ECG manifestations of ARVC, we performed a study aimed at assessment of longitudinal dynamics of the P-wave indices extractable from conventional 12-lead ECG and reported its preliminary results recently.[23] In this study, we included 78 ARVC patients with definite diagnosis (33% females, median age 41 years [IQR 32 to 55 years]) who had available ECGs with P waves from the electronic archives in 3 centers participating in the Nordic ARVC Registry from Denmark and Sweden. All sinus rhythm ECG recordings in the hospital catchment areas starting from the year 1989 were extracted from the regional electronic ECG databases and digitally processed (n = 1291). We studied the progression of ARVC over time based on several P-wave indices, including P-wave duration, PTF-V_1, P-wave area in lead V_1 and V_2, and P-wave frontal axis. Mean values of P-wave indices at diagnosis were compared at 5-year intervals to mean values for the time frame spanning 10 years before and 20 years after ARVC diagnosis.

For the graphical representation of the ARVC progression, we used the fitted Generalized Additive Model (GAM) with cubic splines for all the variables of interest. GAM allows modeling of nonlinear relationships between predictor and response variables by utilizing splines. To account for patient-to-patient variability and balance the data within 1 year, we took a median for each P-wave measurement per patient per year, and then fit GAM.

The mean values of P-wave characteristics 10 years prior to and 20 years after ARVC diagnosis are presented in **Table 12.1**. PTF-V$_1$ increased by 20th year after ARVC diagnosis, and P-wave area in leads V$_1$ and V$_2$ decreased from the time point of 10 years prior to ARVC diagnosis compared to the data at the time of diagnosis and further decreased after ARVC was diagnosed (**Figure 12.2**). P-wave duration and P-wave frontal axis did not change prior to and after ARVC diagnosis. The ECG illustration of P-wave changes during the disease progression is presented in the **Figure 12.3**.

We found P-wave changes that were predominantly related to the evolution of P-wave morphology, but not to changes in P-wave duration during the disease progression.

We observed the decline in P-wave area in leads V$_1$ and V$_2$ starting long before the ARVC diagnosis that likely reflects the right atrial involvement in the disease before ARVC manifestation. The observed changes

possibly indicate that deterioration of atrial myocardium leading to right atrial abnormality takes place in a parallel with progression of RV substrate. Recently, it has been shown that the right atrium undergoes structural changes similar to those of the RV known in ARVC such as a reduction of cardiomyocytes (CMs), the presence of adipocytes, interstitial fibrosis,[24,25] and an increase in size.[26] The gradual reduction of P-wave amplitude in right precordial leads in our study might reflect early right atrial involvement in the disease before ARVC manifestation with gradual development of atrial fibrosis leading to right atrial dilatation. On the other hand, right atrial overload and enlargement might be secondary due to the hemodynamical consequences of the RV contractile dysfunction.[12]

Increased PTF-V$_1$ after 20 years of follow-up found in our study possibly indicate the development of left atrial abnormalities in late stages of the disease. LV involvement in ARVC was demonstrated in 76% of ARVC patients with end-stage disease leading to heart failure.[27,28] LV contractile dysfunc-

TABLE 12.1 Evolution of P-wave indices is presented prior to ARVC diagnosis and during the course of the disease progression. The data are presented as mean ± standard deviation, and variable mean value at each time point is compared to variable mean value at ARVC diagnosis.

YEARS	-10	-5	ARVC DIAGNOSIS	5	10	15	20
PTF-V$_1$, mm*ms	24 ± 11	27 ± 20	24 ± 16	26 ± 22	27 ± 18	31 ± 27*	46 ± 31•
Overall P-wave duration, ms	108 ± 16	112 ± 17	108 ± 18	108 ± 20	105 ± 20	96 ± 17•	109 ± 16
P-wave area in lead V$_1$, µV*ms	24 ± 86#	26 ± 114#	-4 ± 102	-35 ± 126•	-41 ± 118•	-42 ± 119•	-53 ± 99•
P-wave area in lead V$_2$, µV*ms	157 ± 112•	149 ± 133•	90 ± 107	43 ± 138•	20 ± 144•	16 ± 140•	16 ± 114•
P-wave frontal axis, degrees	38 ± 25	43 ± 21	43 ± 26	43 ± 27	40 ± 31	41 ± 26	46 ± 24

PTF-V1 – P-terminal force in lead V$_1$.
*P value < 0.05 in comparison with value at ARVC diagnosis
P value < 0.01 in comparison with value at ARVC diagnosis
• P value < 0.001 in comparison with value at ARVC diagnosis

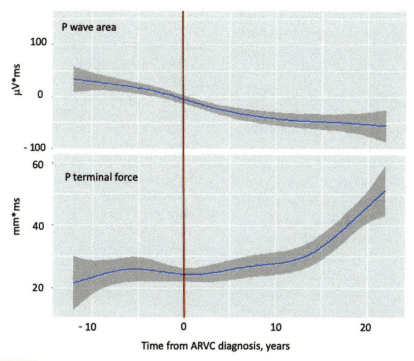

FIGURE 12.2 P-wave area and P-terminal force in lead V$_1$ 10 years prior to ARVC diagnosis and 20 years after. **Blue line** represents the mean, and **gray shadow** is the 95% confidence interval.

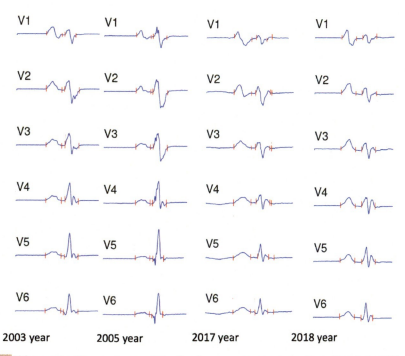

FIGURE 12.3 ECG example of P-wave changes during the disease progression in a patient with definite ARVC.

tion may contribute to left atrial overload, increased stretch, and development of fibrosis in the atrial walls resulting in left atrial remodeling.[13]

Conclusion

AF is common in patients with definite ARVC and is related to the disease severity, thus suggesting AF being an arrhythmic manifestation of this cardiomyopathy. Underlying atrial structural abnormalities provide the substrate for the development of atrial arrhythmias. Atrial myocardial involvement in the disease progression may be studied by analysis of long-term evolution of P-wave indices. According to the preliminary findings from an ongoing registry study, flattening and inversion of P waves in the right precordial leads is observed early in the course of the disease, while electrocardiographic left atrial abnormality appears to be a late manifestation.

References

1. Hoorntje ET, te Rijdt WP, James CA, et al. Arrhythmogenic cardiomyopathy: Pathology, genetics, and concepts in pathogenesis. *Cardiovasc Res.* 2017;113(12):1521–1531.

2. Bourfiss M, te Riele AS, Mast TP, et al. Influence of genotype on structural atrial abnormalities and atrial fibrillation or flutter in arrhythmogenic right ventricular dysplasia/cardiomyopathy. *J Cardiovasc Electrophysiol.* 2016;27(12):1420–1428.

3. Camm CF, James CA, Tichnell C, et al. Prevalence of atrial arrhythmias in arrhythmogenic right ventricular dysplasia/cardiomyopathy. *Heart Rhythm.* 2013;10(11):1661–1668.

4. Chu AF, Zado E, Marchlinski FE. Atrial arrhythmias in patients with arrhythmogenic right ventricular cardiomyopathy/dysplasia and ventricular tachycardia. *Am J Cardiol.* 2010;106(5):720–722.

5. Tonet JL, Castro-Miranda R, Iwa T, Poulain F, Frank R, Fontaine GH. Frequency of supraventricular tachyarrhythmias in arrhythmo-

genic right ventricular dysplasia. *Am J Cardiol.* 1991;67(13):1153.

6. Baturova MA, Haugaa KH, Jensen HK, et al. Atrial fibrillation as a clinical characteristic of arrhythmogenic right ventricular cardiomyopathy: Experience from the nordic ARVC Registry. *Int J Cardiol.* 2020;298:39–43.

7. Gilljam T, Haugaa KH, Jensen HK, et al. Heart transplantation in arrhythmogenic right ventricular cardiomyopathy—Experience from the nordic ARVC Registry. *Int J Cardiol.* 2018;250:201–206.

8. Borgquist R, Haugaa KH, Gilljam T, et al. The diagnostic performance of imaging methods in ARVC using the 2010 Task Force Criteria. *Eur Heart J Cardiovasc Imaging.* 2014;15(11):1219–1225.

9. Marcus FI, McKenna WJ, Sherrill D, et al. Diagnosis of arrhythmogenic right ventricular cardiomyopathy/dysplasia: Proposed modification of the Task Force Criteria. *Circulation.* 2010;121(13):1533–1541.

10. Smith JG, Platonov PG, Hedblad B, Engstrom G, Melander O. Atrial fibrillation in the Malmo diet and cancer study: A study of occurrence, risk factors and diagnostic validity. *Eur J Epidemiol.* 2010;25(2):95–102.

11. Kikuchi N, Yumino D, Shiga T, Suzuki A, Hagiwara N. Long-term prognostic role of the diagnostic criteria for arrhythmogenic right ventricular cardiomyopathy/dysplasia. *JACC Clin Electrophysiol.* 2016;2(1):107–115.

12. Wu L, Guo J, Zheng L, et al. Atrial remodeling and atrial tachyarrhythmias in arrhythmogenic right ventricular cardiomyopathy. *Am J Cardiol.* 2016;118(5):750–753.

13. Corrado D, Basso C, Judge DP. Arrhythmogenic cardiomyopathy. *Circ Res.* 2017;121(7):784–802.

14. Sen-Chowdhry S, Syrris P, McKenna WJ. Role of genetic analysis in the management of patients with arrhythmogenic right ventricular dysplasia/cardiomyopathy. *J Am Coll Cardiol.* 2007;50(19):1813–1821.

15. Mezzano V, Liang Y, Wright AT, et al. Desmosomal junctions are necessary for adult sinus node function. *Cardiovasc Res.* 2016;111(3):274–286.

16. Morimoto S, Sekiguchi M, Okada R, Kasajima T, Hiramitsu S, Yamada K, Mizuno Y. [Two autopsied cases of arrhythmogenic right ventricular dysplasia]. *J Cardiol.* 1990;20(4):1025–1036.

17. Vila J, Pariaut R, Moise NS, Oxford EM, Fox PR, Reynolds CA, Saelinger C. Structural and molecular pathology of the atrium in Boxer arrhythmogenic right ventricular cardiomyopathy. *J Vet Cardiol.* 2017;19(1):57–67.

18. Fox PR, Maron BJ, Basso C, Liu SK, Thiene G. Spontaneously occurring arrhythmogenic right ventricular cardiomyopathy in the domestic cat: A new animal model similar to the human disease. *Circulation.* 2000;102(15):1863–1870.

19. Huo Y, Mitrofanova L, Orshanskaya V, Holmberg P, Holmqvist F, Platonov PG. P-wave characteristics and histological atrial abnormality. *J Electrocardiol.* 2014;47(3):275–280.

20. Tiffany Win T, Ambale Venkatesh B, Volpe GJ, et al. Associations of electrocardiographic P-wave characteristics with left atrial function, and diffuse left ventricular fibrosis defined by cardiac magnetic resonance: The PRIMERI Study. *Heart Rhythm.* 2015;12(1):155–162.

21. Weinsaft JW, Kochav JD, Kim J, et al. P wave area for quantitative electrocardiographic assessment of left atrial remodeling. *PLoS One.* 2014;9(6):e99178.

22. Platonov PG, Christensen AH, Holmqvist F, Carlson J, Haunso S, Svendsen JH. Abnormal atrial activation is common in patients with arrhythmogenic right ventricular cardiomyopathy. *J Electrocardiol.* 2011;44(2):237–241.

23. Baturova MA, Svendsen A, Svendsen JH, Bundgaard H, Sherina V, Carlson J, Platonov PG. Long-term evolution of P wave indices in arrhythmogenic right ventricular cardiomyopathy indicates atrial involvement. *Eur Heart J.* 2018;39(Suppl 1):486.

24. Gehmlich K, Syrris P, Reimann M, et al. Molecular changes in the heart of a severe case of arrhythmogenic right ventricular cardiomyopathy caused by a desmoglein-2 null allele. *Cardiovasc Pathol.* 2012;21(4):275–282.

25. Takemura N, Kono K, Tadokoro K, et al. Right atrial abnormalities in a patient with arrhythmogenic right ventricular cardiomyopathy without ventricular tachycardia. *J Cardiol.* 2008;51(3):205–209.

26. Cardona-Guarache R, Astrom-Aneq M, Oesterle A, et al. Atrial arrhythmias in patients with arrhythmogenic right ventricular cardiomyopathy: Prevalence, echocardiographic predictors, and treatment. *J Cardiovasc Electrophysiol.* 2019;30(10):1801–1810.

27. Basso C, Thiene G, Corrado D, Angelini A, Nava A, Valente M. Arrhythmogenic right ventricular cardiomyopathy: Dysplasia, dystrophy, or myocarditis? *Circulation.* 1996;94(5):983–991.

28. Corrado D, Basso C, Thiene G, et al. Spectrum of clinicopathologic manifestations of arrhythmogenic right ventricular cardiomyopathy/dysplasia: A multicenter study. *J Am Coll Cardiol.* 1997;30(6):1512–1520.

13

Medical Therapy in Arrhythmogenic Right Ventricular Cardiomyopathy

Laura Sommerfeld, MSc; Areej Aljehani, MSc; Manish Kalla, MD; Larissa Fabritz, MD

Introduction

Patients with arrhythmogenic right ventricular cardiomyopathy (ARVC) are commonly advised to make lifestyle adaptations, mainly restriction of sports at the high, competitive level (Class Ic recommendation), even for asymptomatic mutation carriers.[1] This is based on preclinical and clinical data convincingly illustrating that high-level endurance training accelerates the development of ARVC manifesting both as arrhythmic events and as right heart dilatation.[1–6]

Due to the limited number of diagnosed patients, systematic data on therapeutic management and long-term outcome, especially mortality, are still scarce. However, registries and joint efforts from multiple specialized centers across the world have facilitated planned and ongoing randomized studies. This chapter aims to provide an overview of current medical strategies in AVRC as well as ongoing research to identify molecular targets for medical therapy (**Figure 13.1**).

Available Medical Therapies

Traditionally, medical therapy in patients with ARVC was mainly used to prevent ventricular arrhythmias (VAs) and sudden death. *Antiarrhythmic therapy* is currently often used as an adjunct to defibrillation and ablation therapy.[7] A multicenter, retrospective study, including 110 patients, did not show any significant advancement of ventricular tachycardia (VT) in those patients who underwent ablation therapy alone, over those receiving pharmacological therapy.[8] Although heart failure medications, including diuretics, are in clinical use to limit heart failure symptoms in patients with ARVC and heart failure, there is very little evidence on the prognostic effects of these drugs in patients with ARVC. Currently, there is no medical therapy with proven effects on disease progression or prognosis. The need for

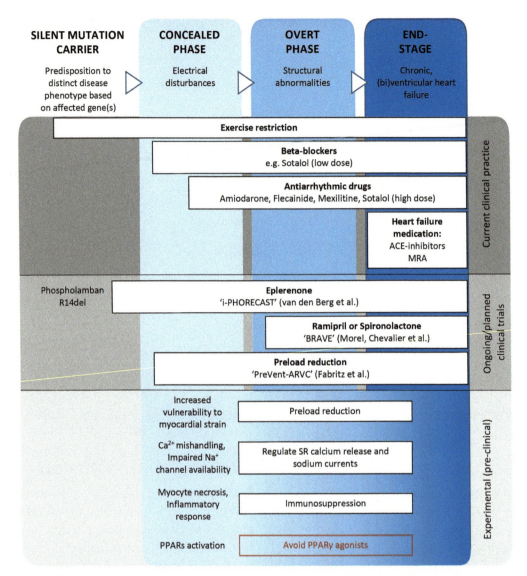

FIGURE 13.1 Summary of current treatment strategies, planned and ongoing clinical trials, and possible new approaches. Abbreviations: ACE, angiotensin-converting enzyme; MRA, mineralocorticoid receptor antagonist; PPAR, peroxisome proliferator-activated receptor; SR, sarcoplasmic reticulum.

new medical therapeutic concepts and clinical studies of novel and traditional concepts therefore remains high.

β-Blockers

As an effective and generally safe antiarrhythmic agent, β-blockers are integrated into the management of ARVC.[1] Their use limits autonomic (adrenergic) dysfunction, which is known to contribute to the disease phenotype as increased adrenergic stimulation in ARVC which facilitates norepinephrine release in the heart. In addition, inhibition of the norepinephrine uptake and subsequent reduction of postsynaptic β-adrenoceptor density have been described.[9–11] Prophylactic use in presymptomatic gene carriers is currently not recommended.[7] Apart from preventing exercise-related catecholaminergic VAs, β-blockers also affect after- and preload.

Load-Reducing Therapy

High preload acutely increases right ventricular (RV) size. Global longitudinal and circumferential strain rates appear to be lower in RV of ARVC patients compared to healthy controls.[12] Decreased wall motion subjects areas in the triangle of dysplasia (RV apex, RV outflow tract [RVOT], tricuspid valve) to high mechanical stress. Reduction of mechanical stress via load reduction has therefore been suggested and was successfully tested in a genetic murine model of ARVC. The combination of nitrates and a diuretic not only prevented exercise-induced RV enlargement, but also reduced occurrence of sustained VTs in hearts of young adult mice.[13] This successful experimental study, employing the decrease of venous return delivered by nitrates and a decrease in systemic blood volume by diuretics, has been translated into a clinical trial plan (PreVent-ARVC). The suggested medical strategy of preload reduction can

be achieved by several drug combinations of choice, including, for example, long-acting nitrates (pentaerithrityl tetranitrate, PETN) or the combination of a thiazide and a potassium-saving diuretic.[14]

ACE Inhibitors, Sartans, and Mineralocorticoid Receptor Antagonists

Angiotensin-converting enzyme (ACE) inhibitors have been considered as part of the therapeutic armamentarium in ARVC, following their effectiveness in left ventricular (LV) failure and considering their effect on preload and afterload. Additionally, angiotensin II is known as an important mediator of cardiac remodeling and can influence matrix metalloproteinase (MMP) transcription.[15] Preliminary results from a small French cohort of ARVC patients suggest that ACE inhibitors can have an effect on extracellular matrix proteins, detected by ratios of MMP9 and its inhibitors tissue inhibitor of metalloproteinase (TIMP)1 and TIMP2 in blood samples. Patients who received β-blockers alone only showed an increase in MMP9/TIMP1 and MMP9/TIMP2 ratios after 1 year, indicating disruption of the extracellular matrix homeostasis. The latter seemed to be stabilized in patients treated with ACE inhibitors on top of β-blockers.[16] This observation led to the design of the BRAVE controlled clinical trial (Counteracting Myocardial Fibrotic Remodelling by Blockade of the Renin-Angiotensin-Aldosterone System in Patients With Arrhythmogenic Right Ventricular Dysplasia, Clinical Trials.gov Identifier: NCT03593317).[16] Commencing in 2021 and conducted in 26 centers in France, this double-blind, parallel, prospective, randomized study will compare disruption of the renin-angiotensin-aldosterone signaling (RAAS) pathway to placebo in a total of 120 participants. It is currently validating whether the trial will utilize spironolactone, an aldosterone inhibitor, instead of the ACE inhibitor ramipril, as originally proposed. The diuretic action of spironolactone is very likely additionally beneficial, as discussed above. Treatment duration for each patient will be 3 years. Primary outcome of the trial is to show reduction in RV deterioration as well as in VA.

The approach of RAAS modulation is also followed up by a Dutch study conducted in a founder mutation cohort of phospholamban R14del carriers (Intervention in PHOspholamban RElated CArdiomyopathy Study, i-PHORECAST, ClinicalTrials.gov Identifier: NCT01857856). Patients with this mutation may develop dilated cardiomyopathy and/or ARVC with early manifestation of cardiac fibrosis (remodeling). The trial will compare the mineralocorticoid receptor antagonist eplerenone to no therapy in mutation carriers with no or only minimal disease signs. The investigators aim to show reduced disease progression and postponed onset of overt disease. With 84 enrolled patients the study is estimated to be completed in 2021.

Antiarrhythmic Drugs

β-blockers and nondihydropyridine calcium-channel blockers (verapamil or diltiazem) have been shown to suppress inducible VAs in patients with ARVC.[17] The nonselective β-blocker and potassium channel blocker sotalol has long been used to improve symptoms in patients with frequent ventricular ectopy or nonsustained VA, and a high efficacy has been reported in a retrospective study.[17,18] Yet, neither sotalol nor other β-blockers have been shown to reduce reentry VA burden in patients with ARVC. When β-blockers, verapamil, or sotalol are ineffective, the antiarrhythmic drug amiodarone is often used, based on expert opinion and some observational data.[1,17,19] Despite relatively high recurrence of VT due to disease progression, ablation therapy is increasingly used (see

elsewhere in this book). The combination of mexiletine and sotalol has been empirically used in some UK centers, often suppressing ectopic activity and arrhythmia sufficiently to avoid such invasive procedures like epicardial ablation in patients with ARVC.

A randomized clinical trial conducted by Kannankeril and colleagues showed that the class Ic antiarrhythmic flecainide on top of β-blocker therapy reduced exercise-induced arrhythmia in catecholaminergic polymorphic ventricular tachycardia (CPVT) patients.[20] Ermakov and colleagues reported positive outcomes from 3 case reports when using a combination of sotalol and flecainide, after insufficient arrhythmia control under monotherapy. Of note, patients presented with an isolated RV disease phenotype and had already received an implantable cardioverter-defibrillator (ICD).[21] Adapting this strategy to treat other patient subgroups is not without risk, not least because the sodium channel blocker flecainide should usually be avoided in structural heart disease. Studies in murine models of ARVC implicated an impairment of functional sodium channel availability based on decreased sodium current density,[22,23] and this observation would not favor medical sodium channel block in ARVC. The ongoing Pilot Randomized Trial With Flecainide in ARVC Patients (ClinicalTrials.gov Identifier: NCT03685149, 2019–2021) investigates the drug's potential to reduce the number of ventricular ectopic beats in ARVC patients who are protected by an ICD.

Anticoagulants

Thromboembolism due to ventricular dilatation, aneurysms, and wall motion abnormalities or even due to atrial fibrillation (AF) might be an accompanying complication of the disease.[24] The annual incidence of thromboembolic events in ARVC in a retrospective study of 126 patients (mean follow-up period of 99 ± 64 months) was reported to be 0.5%.[24]

Oral anticoagulation treatment is recommended for secondary prevention in ARVC patients diagnosed with intracavitary thrombosis or venous systemic thromboembolism. Prophylactic anticoagulation for primary prevention, however, is not recommended.[7]

Developing Medical Therapy to Slow or Prevent Disease Progression

Therapeutic management of ARVC is currently limited to symptomatic treatment that often cannot impede the progressive nature of the disease. Targeting molecular processes taking place during the early, concealed phase prior to clinical manifestation could be a very elegant approach toward active treatment and long-term outcome benefit. Preclinical research suggests that electrophysiological changes can precede the morphological disease phenotype. This was established in a conditional plakophilin-2 knockout mouse model by Kim and colleagues.[25] The group showed increased calcium spark frequency in cardiomyocytes (CMs) and phosphorylation of ryanodine receptors (RyR) at a threonine residue indicated in gating of the channel, specifically in the RV. Normalization of calcium spark frequency back to control levels was achieved via protein kinase C (PKC) inhibition.[25] Widening of the intercellular space due to mechanical junction instability in ARVC might cause dislodgment of signaling molecules like PKC, releasing them from their regulation in their subcellular compartment, causing adverse disease-specific off-target phosphorylation events. The induced abnormal calcium handling during the concealed phase might later on trigger structural abnormalities as observed in the overt phase of ARVC. Suppression of calcium release from the sarcoplasmic reticulum therefore appears to be an attractive therapeutic approach. Some of the beneficial effects of β-blockers might be attributed to restoration of normal RyR2 channel function.[26]

Other pathways indicated in ARVC include Wnt/β-catenin signaling. Plakoglobin (γ-catenin) dislocation from the cardiac intercalated disc has been postulated in ARVC.[27,28] Translocation into the cytoplasm might cause interference with canonical Wnt signaling components, most likely with its structural homologue β-catenin, disturbing homeostasis of the pathway. Downregulated Wnt/β-catenin signaling was, for instance, observed in a transgenic mouse model harboring a human desmoglein-2 nonsense mutation.[29] Alterations in the activity of GSK3β, a core component of the catenin destruction complex, are implicated to contribute to ARVC pathogenesis. Inhibition of GSK3β (and thereby presumably upregulation of Wnt signaling) was beneficial in terms of preventing CM injury and cardiac dysfunction in two genetic mouse and *in vitro* models of the disease.[30] Triggering Wnt signaling, however, is not without risk since increased Wnt activity is found in carcinogenesis of different tissues and knowledge on Wnt activity in other organs of ARVC patients is limited. Tissue-specific drug delivery or identification of cardiac- /CM-specific players of the signaling cascade might lead the way toward safer therapy approaches targeting this pathway.

Canonical Wnt activity alteration in ARVC was also proposed to be caused by abnormal activation of peroxisome proliferator-activated receptors (PPARs), transcriptional regulation factors of fatty acid metabolism.[31,32] Abnormal activation of PPARγ, leading to a decrease in Wnt signaling, might contribute to exaggerated lipogenesis and CM death. Based on this observation, PPARγ agonists like rosiglitazone should be avoided in ARVC patients. Further studies in different models are ongoing.

Necrosis of CMs has been described in ARVC and demonstrated to initiate myocardial injury followed by an inflammatory response of the myocardium.[33] Activation of the immune response has been observed in several ARVC models, based on the presence of antibodies against desmoglein-2.[34] This cardiac immune response includes increased production and release of inflammatory cytokines and exaggerated activation of NFκB. Inhibition of this transcription factor using a small molecule reduced cytokine production and release in vitro, studying human induced pluripotent stem cell-derived cardiomyocytes (hiPSC-CMs), as well as *in vivo*, using a genetic mouse model.[35] This implies immune modulation as a further possible approach.

Treatment strategies and suggested approaches based on preclinical data discussed in this chapter are summarized in Figure 13.1. Clearly, these therapeutic concepts that appear promising in preclinical models require validation and testing in patients with ARVC. Fortunately, such studies have started or are in the planning phase.

Medical Therapy for ARVC: Does One Size Fit All?

This overview is generalized, since observations are derived from preclinical models harboring different ARVC-causing mutations, which translate into diverse disease phenotypes. These are also recognized in patients, as Chen and colleagues very recently established subtype-specific human ARVC pathology based on distinct genetics.[36] Hence, different mutations might require different personalized treatment strategies. Moreover, sex hormone levels seem to influence clinical outcome of the disease.[37] Understanding the molecular basis of these observations will improve medical therapy. The same is true for deciphering disease phase-specific disturbances at molecular level, in particular during the concealed phase, to enable early detection and prevent progression of ARVC to reduce mortality.

References

1. Priori SG, Blomstrom-Lundqvist C, Mazzanti A, et al. ESC guidelines for the management of patients with ventricular arrhythmias and the prevention of sudden cardiac death: The Task Force for the Management of Patients with Ventricular Arrhythmias and the Prevention of Sudden Cardiac Death of the European Society of Cardiology (ESC). Endorsed by: Association for European Paediatric and Congenital Cardiology (AEPC). *Eur Heart J.* 2015;36:2793–2867.

2. Ruwald AC, Marcus F, Estes NA III, et al. Association of competitive and recreational sport participation with cardiac events in patients with arrhythmogenic right ventricular cardiomyopathy: Results from the North American multidisciplinary study of arrhythmogenic right ventricular cardiomyopathy. *Eur Heart J.* 2015;36:1735–1743.

3. James CA, Bhonsale A, Tichnell C, et al. Exercise increases age-related penetrance and arrhythmic risk in arrhythmogenic right ventricular dysplasia/cardiomyopathy-associated desmosomal mutation carriers. *J Am Coll Cardiol.* 2013;62:1290–1297.

4. Kirchhof P, Fabritz L, Zwiener M, et al. Age- and training-dependent development of arrhythmogenic right ventricular cardiomyopathy in heterozygous plakoglobin-deficient mice. *Circulation.* 2006;114:1799–1806.

5. Corrado D, Migliore F, Basso C, Thiene G. Exercise and the risk of sudden cardiac death. *Herz.* 2006;31:553–538.

6. Heidbuchel H, Hoogsteen J, Fagard R, Vanhees L, Ector H, Willems R, Van Lierde J. High prevalence of right ventricular involvement in endurance athletes with ventricular arrhythmias: Role of an electrophysiologic study in risk stratification. *Eur Heart J.* 2003;24:1473–1480.

7. Corrado D, Wichter T, Link MS, et al. Treatment of arrhythmogenic right ventricular cardiomyopathy/dysplasia: An International Task Force consensus statement. *Circulation.* 2015;132:441–453.

8. Mahida S, Venlet J, Saguner AM, et al. Ablation compared with drug therapy for recurrent

ventricular tachycardia in arrhythmogenic right ventricular cardiomyopathy: Results from a multicenter study. *Heart Rhythm.* 2019;16:536–543.

9. Wichter T, Hindricks G, Lerch H, Bartenstein P, Borggrefe M, Schober O, Breithardt G. Regional myocardial sympathetic dysinnervation in arrhythmogenic right ventricular cardiomyopathy: An analysis using 123I-meta-iodobenzylguanidine scintigraphy. *Circulation.* 1994;89:667–683.

10. Paul M, Meyborg M, Boknik P, et al. Autonomic dysfunction in patients with arrhythmogenic right ventricular cardiomyopathy: Biochemical evidence of altered signaling pathways. *Pacing Clin Electrophysiol.* 2014;37:173–178.

11. Wichter T, Schafers M, Rhodes CG, et al. 2000. Abnormalities of cardiac sympathetic innervation in arrhythmogenic right ventricular cardiomyopathy: Quantitative assessment of presynaptic norepinephrine reuptake and postsynaptic beta-adrenergic receptor density with positron emission tomography. *Circulation.* 2000;101:1552–1558.

12. Heermann P, Hedderich DM, Paul M, et al. Biventricular myocardial strain analysis in patients with arrhythmogenic right ventricular cardiomyopathy (ARVC) using cardiovascular magnetic resonance feature tracking. *J Cardiovasc Magn Reson.* 2014;16:75.

13. Fabritz L, Fortmuller L, Yu TY, Paul M, Kirchhof P. Can preload-reducing therapy prevent disease progression in arrhythmogenic right ventricular cardiomyopathy? Experimental evidence and concept for a clinical trial. *Prog Biophys Mol Biol.* 2012;110:340–346.

14. Fabritz L, Hoogendijk MG, Scicluna BP, et al. Load-reducing therapy prevents development of arrhythmogenic right ventricular cardiomyopathy in plakoglobin-deficient mice. *J Am Coll Cardiol.* 2011;57:740–750.

15. Rouet-Benzineb P, Gontero B, Dreyfus P, Lafuma C. Angiotensin II induces nuclear factor-kappa B activation in cultured neonatal rat cardiomyocytes through protein kinase C signaling pathway. *J Mol Cell Cardiol.* 2000;32:1767–1778.

16. Morel E, Manati AW, Nony P, et al. Blockade of the renin-angiotensin-aldosterone system in patients with arrhythmogenic right ventricular dysplasia: A double-blind, multicenter, prospective, randomized, genotype-driven study (BRAVE study). *Clin Cardiol.* 2018;41:300–306.

17. Wichter T, Borggrefe M, Haverkamp W, Chen X, Breithardt G. Efficacy of antiarrhythmic drugs in patients with arrhythmogenic right ventricular disease: Results in patients with inducible and noninducible ventricular tachycardia. *Circulation.* 1992;86:29–37.

18. Wichter T, Paul TM, Eckardt L, Gerdes P, Kirchhof P, Bocker D, Breithardt G. Arrhythmogenic right ventricular cardiomyopathy: Antiarrhythmic drugs, catheter ablation, or ICD? *Herz.* 2005;30:91–101.

19. Marcus GM, Glidden DV, Polonsky B, et al. Efficacy of antiarrhythmic drugs in arrhythmogenic right ventricular cardiomyopathy: A report from the North American ARVC Registry. *J Am Coll Cardiol.* 2009;54:609–615.

20. Kannankeril PJ, Moore JP, Cerrone M, et al. Efficacy of flecainide in the treatment of catecholaminergic polymorphic ventricular tachycardia: A randomized clinical trial. *JAMA Cardiol.* 2017;2:759–766.

21. Ermakov S, Hoffmayer KS, Gerstenfeld EP, Scheinman MM. Combination drug therapy for patients with intractable ventricular tachycardia associated with right ventricular cardiomyopathy. *Pacing Clin Electrophysiol.* 2014;37:90–94.

22. Rizzo S, Lodder EM, Verkerk AO, et al. Intercalated disc abnormalities, reduced Na(+) current density, and conduction slowing in desmoglein-2 mutant mice prior to cardiomyopathic changes. *Cardiovasc Res.* 2012;95:409–418.

23. Cerrone M, Noorman M, Lin X, et al. Sodium current deficit and arrhythmogenesis in a murine model of plakophilin-2 haploinsufficiency. *Cardiovasc Res.* 2012;95:460–468.

24. Wlodarska EK, Wozniak O, Konka M, Rydlewska-Sadowska W, Biederman A, Hoffman P. Thromboembolic complications in patients with arrhythmogenic right ven-

tricular dysplasia/cardiomyopathy. *Europace.* 2006;8:596–600.

25. Kim JC, M. Perez-Hernandez F, Alvarado J, et al. Disruption of Ca(2+)i homeostasis and connexin 43 hemichannel function in the right ventricle precedes overt arrhythmogenic cardiomyopathy in plakophilin-2-deficient mice. *Circulation.* 2019;140:1015–1030.

26. Reiken S, Wehrens XH, Vest JA, et al. Beta-blockers restore calcium release channel function and improve cardiac muscle performance in human heart failure. *Circulation.* 2003;107:2459–2466.

27. Noorman M, Hakim S, Kessler E, et al. Remodeling of the cardiac sodium channel, connexin43, and plakoglobin at the intercalated disk in patients with arrhythmogenic cardiomyopathy. *Heart Rhythm.* 2013;10:412–419.

28. Asimaki A H, Tandri H, Huang MK, et al. A new diagnostic test for arrhythmogenic right ventricular cardiomyopathy. *N Engl J Med.* 2009;360:1075–1084.

29. Calore M, Lorenzon A, Vitiello L, et al. A novel murine model for arrhythmogenic cardiomyopathy points to a pathogenic role of Wnt signaling and miRNA dysregulation. *Cardiovasc Res.* 2019;115:739–751.

30. Chelko SP, Asimaki A, Andersen P, et al. Central role for GSK3beta in the pathogenesis of arrhythmogenic cardiomyopathy. *JCI Insight.* 2016;1(5): e85923.

31. Kim C, Wong J, Wen J, et al. Studying arrhythmogenic right ventricular dysplasia with patient-specific iPSCs. *Nature.* 2013;494:105–110.

32. Djouadi F, Lecarpentier Y, Hebert JL, Charron P, Bastin J, Coirault C. A potential link between peroxisome proliferator-activated receptor signalling and the pathogenesis of arrhythmogenic right ventricular cardiomyopathy. *Cardiovasc Res,* 2009;84:83–90.

33. Pilichou K, Remme CA, Basso C, et al. Myocyte necrosis underlies progressive myocardial dystrophy in mouse dsg2-related arrhythmogenic right ventricular cardiomyopathy. *J Exp Med.* 2009;206:1787–1802.

34. Chatterjee D, Fatah M, Akdis D, et al. An autoantibody identifies arrhythmogenic right ventricular cardiomyopathy and participates in its pathogenesis. *Eur Heart J.* 2018;3(9): 3932–3944.

35. Chelko SP, Asimaki A, Lowenthal J, et al. Therapeutic modulation of the immune response in arrhythmogenic cardiomyopathy. *Circulation.* 2019;140(18):1491–1505.

36. Chen L, Song J, Chen X, et al. A novel genotype-based clinicopathology classification of arrhythmogenic cardiomyopathy provides novel insights into disease progression. *Eur Heart J.* 2019;40:1690–1703.

37. Akdis D, Saguner AM, Shah K, et al. Sex hormones affect outcome in arrhythmogenic right ventricular cardiomyopathy/dysplasia: From a stem cell derived cardiomyocyte-based model to clinical biomarkers of disease outcome. *Eur Heart J.* 2017;38:1498–1508.

14

Role of Catheter Ablation in Arrhythmogenic Right Ventricular Cardiomyopathy

Fabrizio R. Assis, MD; Harikrishna Tandri, MD

Introduction

Ventricular arrhythmia (VA) is the electrical hallmark of arrhythmogenic right ventricular cardiomyopathy (ARVC). Nonuniform fibrofatty infiltration results in a mosaic of healthy myocytes admixed with fibrosis, thus forming a complex, electrically heterogenous substrate. As such, frequent premature ventricular contractions (PVCs) and recurrent ventricular tachycardia (VT) may be seen in all stages of the disease,[1,2] and are associated with a higher risk of sudden cardiac death (SCD).[3] By virtue of this characteristic, the antiarrhythmic management in ARVC involves risk stratification (SCD prevention) and arrhythmia burden reduction (symptom control).

Among the patients at higher risk, implantable cardioverter-defibrillators (ICDs) are the most effective therapy to prevent SCD.

Nevertheless, primary prevention strategy in low-risk patients remains a challenge, and early identification of potential risk factors may play a role in the clinical management.

As VAs are frequent and often symptomatic, antiarrhythmic drugs and β-blockers are commonly used for arrhythmia suppression. Despite this, some patients fail to respond to medical therapy, and catheter ablation has become an attractive option to reduce VT burden and the frequency of ICD shocks.[4,5] Over the past decade, the role of catheter ablation has expanded as novel strategies emerged, especially owing to epicardial ablation, leading to improved long-term results and safer risk profiles. Despite this, VT recurrence is not uncommon, and repeat ablation procedures are still required in a significant number of patients.

In this chapter, we discuss the role of catheter ablation strategies in ARVC.

Catheter Ablation in ARVC

The Substrate

The enhanced sensitivity of diagnostic screening and the technological advances in image assessment and electrical characterization of the substrate led to a better understanding not only of arrhythmogenic substrate distribution in ARVC but also of how it progresses along the course of the disease. Early disease is usually associated with a biventricular scar pattern involving basal inferior and anterior right ventricular (RV) walls, and posterolateral left ventricular (LV) wall, wherein RV apex is commonly spared.[6–8] Initial scarring involves basal inferior RV, particularly the perivalvar region, advancing to the basal anterior segment in moderate disease, and global RV impairment in severe disease (**Figure 14.1**). Low-voltage and fragmented or prolonged-duration electrograms (EGMs), detected within the scar and its borders, and late potentials are typically observed in RV inferobasal regions (perivalvular tricuspid areas) and in different regions of RV anterobasal, anterolateral, and infundibular walls. Although epicardial fat infiltration of the LV posterolateral wall appears to be more frequent than previously recognized, LV dysfunction and arrhythmias originated from that chamber are rare in classic presentations of the disease.

In ARVC, the scarring process is heterogeneous and often transmural, and, as it seems to progress from the epicardium toward the endocardium gradually, epicardial electroanatomic substrate usually predominates over endocardial (**Figure 14.2**).[1,9] The presence of epicardial electrically abnormal areas extending beyond the underlying endocardial electrical substrate and the identification of large epicardial scar with minimal endocardial involvement in early disease have been consistently reported.[4,6,10–12]

Sympathetic Modulation

The strong relationship between the sympathetic nervous system and arrhythmogenesis in ARVC is long recognized.[13–15] Catecholamine challenge during the electrophysiologic assessment of ARVC patients using high-dose isoproterenol infusion has become a common practice in the electrophysiology (EP) lab. Our group originally reported a high degree of association between the morphology of sustained VTs induced during isoproterenol infusion (20 mg/min) and PVCs presented at baseline, wherein mapping and ablation of PVCs eliminated the VTs with the same mor-

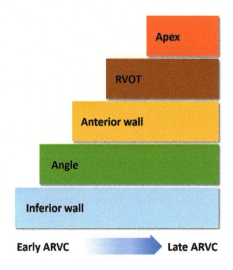

FIGURE 14.1 Scar distribution in different stages of ARVC. Early disease is usually associated with basal involvement, the inferior and lateral (angle) walls (peritricuspid region). As disease progresses, the scar extends through the inferior wall toward the apex and basal anterior wall. In late stages of the disease, the scar extends through lateral and anterior walls, involving the RV outflow tract (RVOT) and, ultimately, the apex.

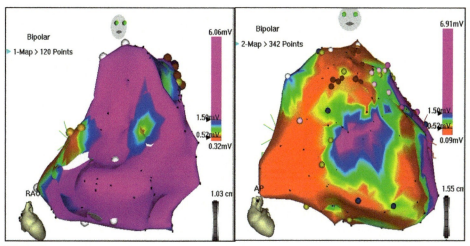

FIGURE 14.2 Scar distribution in ARVC. Shown are the endocardial (**left panel**) and epicardial (**right panel**) maps in sinus rhythm. Small area of perivalvular low voltage was the only endocardial abnormality. Epicardial map (**right panel**) shows extensive scar in the RV base, RVOT, and inferior wall.

phology, all originated from RVOT and RV basal regions (border zones).[16] A high PVC burden during isoproterenol infusion was also associated with shorter VT-free survival after catheter ablation, irrespective of the approach used (endocardial or endo-epicardial),[12] and, although some centers have incorporated systematic PVC elimination into their ablation protocols, the definite value of this strategy still warrants further investigation.

Noninvasive programmed stimulation (NIPS) during mild sedation, preceding general anesthesia/deep sedation induction (sympathetic inhibition), is often helpful to elucidate the clinical target and has been also incorporated as an important step of the electrophysiological assessment in ARVC. A repeat NIPS after ablation (24–48 hours), prior to discharge, has also been performed to guide subsequent management of antiarrhythmic therapy, including early re-intervention or changes in medical therapy.[17]

Endocardial Mapping

Systematic voltage mapping of the endocardial surface should be primarily obtained in sinus rhythm, when feasible, and special attention must be drawn to collecting points in the peritricuspid valve region and anterior RVOT. Confirmation of adequate contact during RV mapping is key as the RV endocardial surface is heavily trabeculated; low-voltage abnormalities may be exaggerated due to the inability to reach the wall, which is especially true when mapping with multielectrode catheters. Contiguous bipolar EGM voltage abnormalities (< 1.5 mV) are registered, and areas of low voltage (< 0.5 mV) represent dense scar, as validated in the literature.[2,18]

At our center, after delineating the endocardial scar, pace mapping is performed to replicate the morphology of clinical VT from the borders of the defined endocardial scar. Documentation of VT morphology by 12-lead electrocardiogram (ECG) is critical, especially when mapping unstable VTs. Areas of long stimulus to QRS and paced morphology similar to clinical VT are marked as possible participants in the VT circuit. VT can be briefly induced, mapped, and entrained from the scar, even if it is not tolerated, in order to get a glimpse of the participation of the endocardial surface in the VT circuit.

In the early stages of the disease, endocardial scar may be minimal or not even detectable at bipolar voltage mapping. Herein, obtaining a unipolar voltage mapping may provide valuable information regarding both presence and extension of epicardial scar, given the recognized association between unipolar low-voltage endocardium areas (< 5.5 mV) and epicardial scar.[11,19,20] Prior failed endocardial ablation, VT ECG morphology, identification of islands of epicardial scar at cardiac imaging, limited electroanatomic substrate in the endocardium, lack of a good pace map while stimulating potential target areas along the endocardial surface, and failure to eliminate the VT after endocardial mapping and ablation all collectively favor the value of epicardial assessment. Nevertheless, these findings should not be considered independently as none of them have been individually linked to better acute- or long-term outcomes.

Epicardial Access

The use of epicardial access has consistently increased in the past decade and accounts for up to two-thirds of procedures reported.[5] The electrophysiologist should be fully aware of the anatomical nuances (e.g., coronary anatomy, fat distribution) and associated risks of accessing the pericardial space. In order to minimize such risks, preprocedural imaging should be obtained for all patients to define thoracic anatomy and anticipate local anatomical constraints that might complicate or obviate access or even catheter manipulation inside the pericardial space. Anticoagulation must be held before the procedure following drug-specific instructions.

In our institution, we use an anterior approach to obtain epicardial access in all patients undergoing epicardial ablation (**Figure 14.3**). Epidural introducer needle is inserted through a small subxiphoid incision at a 20-degree angle; under biplane fluoroscopy guidance, the needle is carefully advanced through a shallow path toward the anterior aspect of the RV silhouette. Once the needle has approached the pericardium, a small amount of contrast is injected to confirm pericardium tenting. The needle is then further advanced, and the pericardium space is accessed. Additional contrast is injected to reassure location, which is followed by insertion of a 0.035-in Bentson J-tipped floppy guidewire (Cook Medical, Bloomington, IN) into the pericardial space. The guidewire should freely travel inside the pericardial space, wrapping around the heart across multiple chambers. After access is established and confirmed, a long deflectable sheath is advanced over the guidewire into the pericardial space.[21] In the supine position, the pericardial fluid tends to be displaced anteriorly, favoring safer access to anterior and basal regions of both ventricles, as it avoids the atrioventricular (AV) groove and thus reduces the odds of vascular injury. Also, the shallow path across thoraco-abdominal transition reduces the risk of hepatic or bowel laceration.

Epicardial Mapping and Ablation

The existence of complex subepicardial and midmyocardial circuits associated with the inability to generate lesions deep enough to eliminate them from the endocardial surface is considered one of the central reasons leading to failed endocardial-only ablation.[22] Early recognition of subepicardial circuits is key for reducing procedural time and delineating a successful ablation strategy (see the section *Endocardial Mapping*). Detailed, high-density biventricular epicardium mapping allows for an extensive assessment of scar and its borders, wherein voltage > 1.0 mV identifies normal myocardium.[23] The unique pattern of scar distribution in the peritricuspid region, especially in the basal inferior RV, results in reentrant circuits

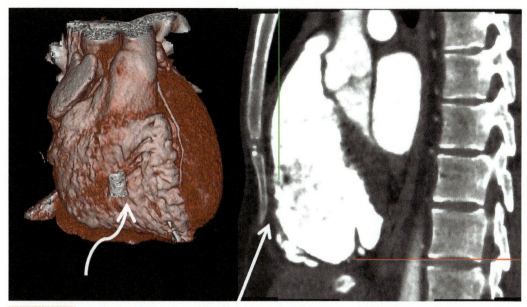

FIGURE 14.3 Anterior epicardial access: CT scan in coronal and sagittal views shows the trajectory of anterior epicardial access in ARVC.

and hence superior axis VTs with late precordial transition in V_4 and V_5. Late potentials well after the QRS are the rule in this region, and detailed pace mapping in this scar is often valuable in determining potential exit sites of reentrant VTs. Multiple VT morphologies often share the same circuit (different exit sites), and channels in the basal scar are commonly involved.

Inferior axis VTs are most often related to the epicardial scar in the anterior RVOT. Careful annotation of late potentials and recording the EGMs that represent the AV groove are critical for ablation planning in ARVC. Epicardial scar often extends to the AV groove, and ablation in this region also carries a risk of injury to the right coronary artery. Further, the AV groove hosts a variable but often significant amount of epicardial fat, which may affect mapping quality and ablation results. This is particularly important in ARVC patients as most VT circuits are located along the basal RV (perivalvar region) and basal lateral wall, which in turn constitute primary sites of epicardial fat distribution.

In addition, the presence of fibrofatty replacement resultant from the ARVC scarring process further contributes to fat deposition in those same areas. While the presence of late potentials seems to be highly specific for scar (99%) in areas with fat deposition, bipolar low-voltage signals alone cannot differentiate epicardial scar from fat. Unipolar voltage maps, however, appear not to be impaired by fat distribution and may be superior in identifying scar swathed by fat.[24] Large isthmuses are often found in moderate-severe ARVC, and linear lesions through isthmus or diastolic pathway, extended to valvular anatomic boundaries, scar, or preserved myocardium, should be performed to achieve efficient substrate modification.

Noninducibility during programmed stimulation after the ablation has been associated with better arrhythmia, particularly when performed under isoproterenol sensibilization.[25–28] Mapping and systematic ablation of PVCs are also undertaken at some centers; however, the effect of this strategy on overall outcomes remains unclear.

Complications

The expansion of the number of epicardial ablation procedures performed in ARVC patients led to a slight increase in complication rates when compared to endocardial-only ablation procedures. Pericarditis without pericardial effusion is the most frequent complication, reported in up to 20%–30% of patients.[29,30] Major complications occur in 4%–10% of patients and often include pericardial tamponade (most common), persistent bleeding, extensive pericardial inflammation, coronary injury, and acute myocardial infarction.[29,31,32]

In a study including 100 consecutive epicardial procedures, our group reported the feasibility and safety of using an anterior approach to access the pericardium space. In this series, successful epicardial access was obtained in all patients without significant pericardial bleeding (> 80 mL), RV puncture, or need for emergent cardiac surgery. Although self-limited pericarditis was seen in all patients in this series, only 2 subjects required colchicine at discharge.[21]

Outcomes

Overall, a combined endo-epicardial approach has been associated with better long-term results, especially in patients who failed a prior endocardial-only ablation. Existent data on VT ablation outcomes are largely heterogenous, with VT-free survival rates ranging between 35% and 89% (**Table 14.1**). Although existent data suggest a potential benefit of an early epicardial approach, whether its systematic application as a first-line strategy yields additional benefit is still to be determined. In a study investigating the role of an adjuvant epicardial catheter ablation, a combined approach was only performed in cases of recurrent VT or persistent VT inducibility after endocardial ablation; endo-epicardial ablation was required in 63% of patients, with an overall VT-free survival rate of 71% (mean follow-up of 56 months).[5] This was later corroborated by other centers supporting a stepwise approach for the use of epicardial procedures.[33,34] In our institution, while employing a similar strategy, approximately two-thirds of patients required epicardial ablation during the first ablation procedure, and those patients who underwent an endocardial-only intervention showed similar VT-free or ICD shocks survival rates when comparing endocardial vs. epicardial strategies (unpublished data). A high number of induced VTs during the procedure and failure to deem the patient noninducible after ablation (unsuccessful procedure) have been associated with VT recurrence during the follow-up.

It is worth mentioning that, besides the improved short- and long-term VT-free outcomes, VT ablation also reduces the need for antiarrhythmic drugs and ICD interventions. Though repeat procedures are not rare, the value of multiple procedures is still debatable. Although early studies have failed to prove the existence of a cumulative benefit on VT-free survival rates associated with repeat procedures,[4,35] recent data seem to suggest a further reduction of VA burden after subsequent ablations.[36]

Early data has shown neuraxial modulation with bilateral cardiac sympathetic denervation (BCSD) as a valid and safe adjunctive strategy in ARVC patients who failed ablation. In our experience, BCSD significantly reduced the VT burden, the number of ICD shocks, and the need for antiarrhythmic medications in patients who failed a prior VT ablation procedure.[37] This is especially true in young patients with rapid adrenergically mediated VAs and a high burden of polymorphic PVCs. Nevertheless, further investigation is necessary to define the optimal timing of BCSD and whether different stages of the disease equally benefit from the procedure.

TABLE 14.1 Long-term results of catheter ablation for VT in ARVC

STUDY	YEAR	TARGET SURFACE	FOLLOW-UP DURATION	LONG-TERM RESULTS
Marchlinski et al.[38]	2004	Endo (1 Epi – RBBB VT)	27 ± 22 m	**VT-free survival:** 89%
Verma et al.[39]	2005	Endo	37 m (25 – 44 m)	**VT recurrence:** 23% (1 y), 27% (2 y), and 47% (3 y)
Dalal et al.[35]	2007	Endo No EAM: 79%	32 ± 36 m	**Cumulative VT-free survival:** 75% (1.5 m), 50% (5 m), and 25% (14 m) **Cumulative incidence of VT recurrence:** 64% (1 y), 75% (2 y), and 91% (3 y)
Garcia et al.[10]	2009	Endo + Epi	18 ± 13 m	**VT-free survival (last ablation):** 77%
Bai et al.[12]	2011	Endo: 47% Endo + Epi: 53%	3 y (overall) 1224 ± 310 d (Endo) 1175 ± 112 d (Epi)	**Freedom from VAs or ICD therapy (Endo):** 52.2% **Freedom from VAs or ICD therapy (Endo + Epi):** 84.6%
Berruezo et al.[40]	2012	Endo + Epi: (Scar dechanneling)	11 m	**VT-free survival:** 91% (midterm follow-up)
Philips et al.[41]	2012	EAM: 69% procedures Endo: 85% Endo + Epi: 9% Epi: 6%	88 ± 66 m	**VT-free survival (single procedure):** 47% (1 y), 31% (2 y), 21% (5 y), and 15% (10 y) **VT-free survival (after a single Endo catheter ablation):** 45% (1 y), 29% (2 y), and 19% (5 y) **VT-free survival (after a single Epi catheter ablation):** 64% (1 y), 45% (2 y), and 45% (5 y)
Santangeli et al.[42]	2015	Endo: 37% Endo + Epi (adjuvant): 63%	56 ± 44 m	**VT-free survival:** 71%
Philips et al.[43]	2015	Endo + Epi: 40% Epi: 60%	19.7 ± 11.7 m	**VT-free survival:** 83% (6m), 76% (12 m), and 70% (24 m)
Wei et al.[44]	2017	Endo: 74% Epi: 26%	71.4 ± 45.7 m	**VT-free survival after a single catheter ablation:** 37.5% **VT-free survival after last catheter ablation:** 56.3% Acute procedural success was associated with longer VT-free survival
Berruezo et al.[20]	2017	Endo + Epi: (1st ablation)	32.2 ± 21.8 m	**VT-recurrence (end of follow-up):** 26.8% Left-dominant AC associated with a higher risk of VT recurrence Bi/Uni-LVA ratio > 0.23 was associated with limited epicardial substrate

(continued)

TABLE 14.1 *(continued)*

STUDY	YEAR	TARGET SURFACE	FOLLOW-UP DURATION	LONG-TERM RESULTS
Mussigbrodt et al.[33]	2017	Endo: 100% Epi (adjuvant): 49%	31.1 ± 27.4 m	**VT-free survival (Endo-only):** 56.5% **VT-free survival (Endo + Epi):** 59.1% Inducibility-guided ablation strategy yielded similar long-term results irrespective of the approach (Endo or Endo + Epi)
Laredo et al.[45]	2019	Epi: 17%	3.9 y (1 m – 10 y)	**ES-free survival:** 100% (1 y), 85% (5 y) **VT-free survival:** 77% (1 y), 66% (5 y)
Mathew et al.[34]	2019	Endo: 56% Epi + Endo: 31% Epi: 13%	50.8 (18.6–99.2 m)	**VT/VF-free survival after index catheter ablation:** 36% (end of follow-up) **VT/VF-free survival after multiple catheter ablation:** 63% (1 y), 45% (5 y) 36% of patients underwent only endocardial catheter ablation
Mahida et al.[46]	2019	Endo: 47% Epi: 53%	3 ± 4.2 y	**VT-free survival after a single catheter ablation:** 35% (3 y) **VT-free survival after the last catheter ablation:** 56% (3 y) **VT-free survival after the last catheter ablation (at least one Endo-Epi):** 71% (3 y) **VT-free survival after the last catheter ablation (Endo-only):** 47% (3 y) No difference in VT-free survival was observed when comparing a single catheter ablation vs. AAD escalation
Christiansen et al.[47]	2020	Endo: 84% Epi: 16%	7.9 (IQR 4.9–12.5 y)	**VT-free survival after first-time catheter ablation:** 25% Young age, use of several AAD, and VT inducibility after the procedure were associated with unfavorable outcomes
Liang et al.[48]	2020	Endo: 96% Epi: 4%	46.3 ± 40.7 m	**VT-free survival after catheter ablation:** 56.7% **VT-free survival after the last catheter ablation:** 78.1% ≥ 3 induced VTs were associated with VT recurrence

Abbreviation: ES, electrical storm.

References

1. Basso C, Thiene G, Corrado D, Angelini A, Nava A, Valente M. Arrhythmogenic right ventricular cardiomyopathy: Dysplasia, dystrophy, or myocarditis? *Circulation.* 1996;94:983–991.

2. Marchlinski FE. Electroanatomic substrate and outcome of catheter ablative therapy for ventricular tachycardia in setting of right ventricular cardiomyopathy. *Circulation.* 2004;110:2293–2298.

3. Calkins H, Corrado D, Marcus F. Risk stratification in arrhythmogenic right ventricular cardiomyopathy. *Circulation.* 2017;136:2068–2082.

4. Philips B, te Riele AS, Sawant A, et al. Outcomes and ventricular tachycardia recurrence characteristics after epicardial ablation of ventricular tachycardia in arrhythmogenic right ventricular dysplasia/cardiomyopathy. *Heart Rhythm.* 2015;12:716–725.

5. Santangeli P, Zado ES, Supple GE, et al. Long-term outcome with catheter ablation of ventricular tachycardia in patients with arrhythmogenic right ventricular cardiomyopathy. *Circ Arrhythm Electrophysiol.* 2015;8:1413–1421.

6. te Riele AS, James CA, Philips B, et al. Mutation-positive arrhythmogenic right ventricular dysplasia/cardiomyopathy: The triangle of dysplasia displaced. *J Cardiovasc Electrophysiol.* 2013;24:1311–1320.

7. Sen-Chowdhry S, Syrris P, Ward D, Asimaki A, Sevdalis E, McKenna WJ. Clinical and genetic characterization of families with arrhythmogenic right ventricular dysplasia/cardiomyopathy provides novel insights into patterns of disease expression. *Circulation.* 2007;115:1710–1720.

8. Bauce B, Basso C, Rampazzo A, et al. Clinical profile of four families with arrhythmogenic right ventricular cardiomyopathy caused by dominant desmoplakin mutations. *Eur Heart J.* 2005;26:1666–1675.

9. Corrado D, Basso C, Thiene G, et al. Spectrum of clinicopathologic manifestations of arrhythmogenic right ventricular cardiomyopathy/dysplasia: A multicenter study. *J Am Coll Cardiol.* 1997;30:1512–1520.

10. Garcia FC, Bazan V, Zado ES, Ren J-F, Marchlinski FE. Epicardial substrate and outcome with epicardial ablation of ventricular tachycardia in arrhythmogenic right ventricular cardiomyopathy/dysplasia. *Circulation.* 2009;120:366–375.

11. Polin GM, Haqqani H, Tzou W, et al. Endocardial unipolar voltage mapping to identify epicardial substrate in arrhythmogenic right ventricular cardiomyopathy/dysplasia. *Heart Rhythm.* 2011;8:76–83.

12. Bai R, Di Biase L, Shivkumar K, et al. Ablation of ventricular arrhythmias in arrhythmogenic right ventricular dysplasia/cardiomyopathy: Arrhythmia-free survival after endo-epicardial substrate based mapping and ablation. *Circ Arrhythm Electrophysiol.* 2011;4:478–485.

13. Wichter T, Hindricks G, Lerch H, et al. Regional myocardial sympathetic dysinnervation in arrhythmogenic right ventricular cardiomyopathy. An analysis using 123I-meta-iodobenzylguanidine scintigraphy. *Circulation.* 1994;89:667–683.

14. Corrado D, Basso C, Rizzoli G, Schiavon M, Thiene G. Does sports activity enhance the risk of sudden death in adolescents and young adults? *J Am Coll Cardiol.* 2003;42:1959–1963.

15. James CA, Bhonsale A, Tichnell C, et al. Exercise increases age-related penetrance and arrhythmic risk in arrhythmogenic right ventricular dysplasia/cardiomyopathy–associated desmosomal mutation carriers. *J Am Coll Cardiol.* 2013;62:1290–1297.

16. Philips B, Madhavan S, James C, et al. High prevalence of catecholamine-facilitated focal ventricular tachycardia in patients with arrhythmogenic right ventricular dysplasia/cardiomyopathy. *Circ Arrhythm Electrophysiol.* 2013;6:160–166.

17. Frankel DS, Mountantonakis SE, Zado ES, et al. Noninvasive programmed ventricular stimulation early after ventricular tachycardia ablation to predict risk of late recurrence. *J J Am Coll Cardiol.* 2012;59:1529–1535.

18. Hsia HH, Callans DJ, Marchlinski FE. Characterization of endocardial electrophysiologi-

cal substrate in patients with nonischemic cardiomyopathy and monomorphic ventricular tachycardia. *Circulation.* 2003;108:704–710.

19. Tschabrunn CM, Santangeli P, Frankel DS, Zado ES, Callans DJ, Marchlinski FE. Isolated epicardial electrogram abnormalities in arrhythmogenic right ventricular cardiomyopathy (ARVC): Implications for diagnosis and treatment. *Circulation.* 2019;140:A15876-A.

20. Berruezo A, Acosta J, Fernandez-Armenta J, et al. Safety, long-term outcomes and predictors of recurrence after first-line combined endo-epicardial ventricular tachycardia substrate ablation in arrhythmogenic cardiomyopathy. Impact of arrhythmic substrate distribution pattern: A prospective multicentre study. *Europace.* 2017;19:607–616.

21. Keramati AR, DeMazumder D, Misra S, et al. Anterior pericardial access to facilitate electrophysiology study and catheter ablation of ventricular arrhythmias: A single tertiary center experience. *J Cardiovasc Electrophysiol.* 2017;28:1189–1195.

22. Haqqani HM, Tschabrunn CM, Betensky BP, et al. Layered activation of epicardial scar in arrhythmogenic right ventricular dysplasia: Possible substrate for confined epicardial circuits. *Circ Arrhythm Electrophysiol.* 2012;5:796–803.

23. Cano O, Hutchinson M, Lin D, et al. Electro-anatomic substrate and ablation outcome for suspected epicardial ventricular tachycardia in left ventricular nonischemic cardiomyopathy. *J Am Coll Cardiol.* 2009;54:799–808.

24. van Taxis CFvH, Wijnmaalen AP, Piers SR, van der Geest RJ, Schalij MJ, Zeppenfeld K. Real-time integration of MDCT-derived coronary anatomy and epicardial fat: Impact on epicardial electroanatomic mapping and ablation for ventricular arrhythmias. *JACC Cardiovasc Imaging.* 2013;6:42–52.

25. Calkins H, Epstein A, Packer D, et al. Catheter ablation of ventricular tachycardia in patients with structural heart disease using cooled radiofrequency energy: Results of a prospective multicenter study. *J Am Coll Cardiol.* 2000;35:1905–1914.

26. Kottkamp H, Hindricks G, Chen X, et al. Radiofrequency catheter ablation of sustained ventricular tachycardia in idiopathic dilated cardiomyopathy. *Circulation.* 1995;92:1159–1168.

27. Soejima K, Stevenson WG, Sapp JL, Selwyn AP, Couper G, Epstein LM. Endocardial and epicardial radiofrequency ablation of ventricular tachycardia associated with dilated cardiomyopathy: The importance of low-voltage scars. *J Am Coll Cardiol.* 2004;43:1834–1842.

28. Stevenson WG, Wilber DJ, Natale A, et al. Irrigated radiofrequency catheter ablation guided by electroanatomic mapping for recurrent ventricular tachycardia after myocardial infarction: The multicenter thermocool ventricular tachycardia ablation trial. *Circulation.* 2008;118:2773–2782.

29. Della Bella P, Brugada J, Zeppenfeld K, et al. Epicardial ablation for ventricular tachycardia: A European multicenter study. *Circ Arrhythm Electrophysiol.* 2011;4:653–659.

30. Sosa E, Scanavacca M. Epicardial approach to catheter ablation of ventricular tachycardia. *Catheter Ablation of Cardiac Arrhythmias*, 2nd edition. Boston, MA: Elsevier; 2011:560–573.

31. Sacher F, Roberts-Thomson K, Maury P, et al. Epicardial ventricular tachycardia ablation a multicenter safety study. *J Am Coll Cardiol.* 2010;55:2366–2372.

32. Tung R, Michowitz Y, Yu R, et al. Epicardial ablation of ventricular tachycardia: An institutional experience of safety and efficacy. *Heart Rhythm.* 2013;10:490–498.

33. Mussigbrodt A, Efimova E, Knopp H, et al. Should all patients with arrhythmogenic right ventricular dysplasia/cardiomyopathy undergo epicardial catheter ablation? *J Interv Card Electrophysiol.* 2017;48:193–199.

34. Mathew S, Saguner AM, Schenker N, et al. Catheter ablation of ventricular tachycardia in patients with arrhythmogenic right ventricular cardiomyopathy/dysplasia: A sequential approach. *J Am Heart Assoc.* 2019;8(5):e010365.

35. Dalal D, Jain R, Tandri H, et al. Long-term efficacy of catheter ablation of ventricular

tachycardia in patients with arrhythmogenic right ventricular dysplasia/cardiomyopathy. *J Am Col Cardiolol.* 2007;50:432–440.

36. Tzou WS, Tung R, Frankel DS, et al. Outcomes after repeat ablation of ventricular tachycardia in structural heart disease: An analysis from the International VT Ablation Center Collaborative Group. *Heart Rhythm.* 2017;14:991–997.

37. Assis FR, Krishnan A, Zhou X, et al. Cardiac sympathectomy for refractory ventricular tachycardia in arrhythmogenic right ventricular cardiomyopathy. *Heart Rhythm.* 2019;16(7):1003–1010.

38. Marchlinski FE, Zado E, Dixit S, et al. Electroanatomic substrate and outcome of catheter ablative therapy for ventricular tachycardia in setting of right ventricular cardiomyopathy. *Circulation.* 2004;110:2293–2298.

39. Verma A, Kilicaslan F, Schweikert RA, et al. Short-and long-term success of substrate-based mapping and ablation of ventricular tachycardia in arrhythmogenic right ventricular dysplasia. *Circulation.* 2005;111:3209–3216.

40. Berruezo A, Fernández-Armenta J, Mont L, et al. Combined endocardial and epicardial catheter ablation in arrhythmogenic right ventricular dysplasia incorporating scar dechanneling technique. *Circ Arrhythm Electrophysiol.* 2012;5:111–121.

41. Philips B, Madhavan S, James C, et al. Outcomes of catheter ablation of ventricular tachycardia in arrhythmogenic right ventricular dysplasia/cardiomyopathy. *Circ Arrhythm Electrophysiol.* 2012;5:499–505.

42. Santangeli P, Zado ES, Supple GE, et al. Long-term outcome with catheter ablation of ventricular tachycardia in patients with arrhythmogenic right ventricular cardiomyopathy. *Circ Arrhythm Electrophysiol.* 2015;8:1413–1421.

43. Philips B, te Riele A, Sawant A, et al. Outcomes and VT recurrence characteristics after epicardial ablation of ventricular tachycardia in arrhythmogenic right ventricular dysplasia/cardiomyopathy. *Heart Rhythm.* 2015;12:716–725.

44. Wei W, Liao H, Xue Y, et al. Long-term outcomes of radio-frequency catheter ablation on ventricular tachycardias due to arrhythmogenic right ventricular cardiomyopathy: A single center experience. *PLoS One* 2017;12:e0169863.

45. Laredo M, Oliveira Da Silva L, Extramiana F, et al. Catheter ablation of electrical storm in patients with arrhythmogenic right ventricular cardiomyopathy. *Heart Rhythm.* 2020;17(1):41–48.

46. Mahida S, Venlet J, Saguner AM, et al. Ablation compared with drug therapy for recurrent ventricular tachycardia in arrhythmogenic right ventricular cardiomyopathy: Results from a multicenter study. *Heart Rhythm.* 2019;16:536–543.

47. Christiansen MK, Haugaa KH, Svensson A, et al. Incidence, predictors, and success of ventricular tachycardia catheter ablation in arrhythmogenic right ventricular cardiomyopathy (from the Nordic ARVC Registry). *Am J Cardiol.* 2020;125:803–811.

48. Liang E, Wu L, Fan S, et al. Catheter ablation of arrhythmogenic right ventricular cardiomyopathy ventricular tachycardia: 18-year experience in 284 patients. *EP Europace* 2020;22: 806–812.

Arrhythmogenic Right Ventricular Cardiomyopathy Research: Better Together

Anneline S.J.M. te Riele, MD, PhD; Laurens P. Bosman, MD; Julia Cadrin-Tourigny, MD; Cynthia A. James, PhD, ScM

Introduction

Following the seminal work of Marcus and colleagues describing arrhythmogenic right ventricular cardiomyopathy (ARVC) in the modern scientific literature,[1] remarkable progress has been made in our understanding of the genetic basis, clinical course, diagnosis, and management of this intriguing disease. Research from local and national registries has been critically important to this progress. However, several challenges associated with the epidemiology and natural history of the disease have confronted clinical registry-based ARVC research. First, with an estimated prevalence of 1 in 2000 to 5000 individuals, the disease is relatively rare and research studies are often underpowered.[2] Second, ARVC has wide clinical variability, which limits extrapolation of results.[3] Third, the incomplete penetrance and variable expressivity of ARVC suggest a strong role for genetic and environmental modifiers.[4]

While this provides opportunities for personalized management based on genotype and lifestyle, it also requires larger samples sizes to adequately account for these effects. Fourth, a significant proportion of ARVC patients present with sudden cardiac death (SCD), which leads to survival bias (i.e., research studies only include subjects presenting alive with a "less severe" phenotype) that is virtually impossible to correct for.[5] Finally, since ARVC is a genetic disease, at-risk relatives who may not (yet) have disease expression also require study but need even larger sample sizes given their less frequent events. Strong research on the pathogenesis, natural history, and treatment of this disease is therefore both timely and important.

To overcome these challenges, the ARVC community has recognized that collaborative efforts are key. Collaboration facilitates both scientific exchange and assembly of cohorts large enough for adequate statistical power. In this chapter, we describe the development, structure, and approach to enrollment and follow-up of two large ARVC Registries: the Johns Hopkins ARVC Registry and the Netherlands Arrhythmogenic Cardiomyopathy (ACM) Registry. We also describe our experience integrating data between the registries and highlight several scientific successes that resulted not only from increased sample size and statistical power but also from intellectual exchange among our programs. This chapter ends with a vision for a nascent collaborative ARVC clinical research network to address the complex challenges of improving care for ARVC patients and families.

Challenges and Achievements After 20 Years of a Large Registry: The North American Experience

History of the Registry

The Johns Hopkins ARVD/C Program (www.arvd.com) was established in 1999 through the combined efforts of several families and a team of cardiologists. When the program was established, we identified 3 primary goals. The first goal was to provide education for patients, families, and physicians about ARVC. A second goal was to facilitate the evaluation and management of patients with known or suspected ARVC and at-risk relatives. The third, and perhaps most important, goal was to provide new knowledge about ARVC with the ultimate goal to use these data to help cure and/or prevent ARVC. The prospective Johns Hopkins ARVC Registry was established in 2000 as our primary clinical research tool to facilitate this effort.

Structure of the Registry

Individuals eligible to join the Johns Hopkins ARVC Registry include those with a presumptive clinical diagnosis of ARVC in addition to patients with a confirmed diagnosis based on the 2010 Task Force Criteria (TFC)[6] and those at risk based on their genotype or family history (or both). The broad enrollment criteria allow data from the registry to be used to evaluate diagnostic approaches and identify ARVC mimics in addition to conducting studies characterizing ARVC patients and families. To date, the registry has enrolled 1813 individuals. As shown in **Table 15.1**, slightly more than half (N = 982) of participants are either definite ARVC patients per the 2010 TFC or at risk based on their family history and/or genotype.

To build the registry, it was necessary to overcome not only the challenges associated with the relative rarity of ARVC compounded by sudden death presentation and underdiagnosis but also the decentralized structure of the U.S. healthcare system. While patients often seek an expert opinion at our center, many also require ongoing local care and/or are limited by their insurance networks. To respond to this challenge, the Johns Hopkins ARVC Registry research cohort has been built by prioritizing outreach and participant engagement. This approach allows us to enroll ARVC patients and families from across North America, including those not followed at our center.

Registry enrollment and follow-up are led by dedicated program genetic counselors. Participants with definite ARVC or at risk based on genotype or family history are invited to submit a DNA sample and complete questionnaires/interviews to document exercise history, family history, pregnancy history, and psychosocial adaptation. Relationships with participants are strengthened by an annual free patient-family meeting held each spring to bring families together for education, for mutual support, and to participate in research.[7]

The registry is approved by the Johns Hopkins Medicine Institutional Review Board (NA_00041248). Curated data are maintained in a REDCap database (Vanderbilt University, Nashville, TN) linked to a university-supported networked "virtual file cabinet"

TABLE 15.1 Characteristics of ARVC patients and at-risk individuals enrolled in the Johns Hopkins and Netherlands ARVC/ACM Registries are presented.

	JOHNS HOPKINS *N* = 982 (CASES AND AT-RISK)	NETHERLANDS *N* = 911 (CASES AND AT-RISK)
Index patients	502 (51%)	238 (26%)
Male	498 (51%)	475 (52%)
Mutation carrier	560 (57%)	493 (54%)
- PKP2	418 (75% of mutations)	401 (81% of mutations)
- PLN	11 (2%)	68 (14%)
- DSG2	35 (6%)	12 (2%)
- DSP	78 (14%)	8 (2%)
- Other	18 (3%)	4 (1%)
Definite ARVC diagnosis	562 (57%)	420 (46%)
Median follow-up	5.2 years	7.9 years

(OnBase), which allows linked viewing of raw documents (electrocardiogram [ECG], Holter, clinic notes, etc.). This system has recently been updated and aligned with the Netherlands REDCap database, described below. This upgrade was made possible through financial support of our university via selection of ARVC as a Precision Medicine Center of Excellence (see www.hopkinsmedicine.org /inhealth/precision-medicine-centers/arvc/).

Research Foci and Successes

Initial research goals of the Johns Hopkins ARVD/C Program included improving ARVC diagnosis, defining natural history, identifying ARVC genes, and defining genotype–phenotype relationships. Considerable progress has been achieved in each area. Early successes included the first description of the natural history of ARVC in an American cohort,[8] publications defining the prevalence and penetrance of *PKP2* variants in our population,[9,10] identification of *DSG2* as an ARVC gene,[11] and numerous publications defining best practices for imaging in ARVC diagnosis.[12–15] Data from these early studies were used to inform revision of the ARVC diagnostic criteria in 2010.[6]

More recently, our clinical and translational research focus has turned toward defining the predictors and modifiers of outcomes among both patients and their at-risk relatives so as to facilitate evidence-based, personalized management.

Influence of Exercise

We have extensively examined the role of aerobic exercise on outcomes in ARVC patients and relatives. Based on clinical, genetic, and exercise history data in the registry, we have established that aerobic exercise increases age-related penetrance, arrhythmic risk, and likelihood of heart failure in ARVC patients and family members with desmosomal mutations.[16,17] We have also shown that gene-elusive ARVC patients are disproportionately high-level athletes and have a paucity of family history, suggesting this cohort of patients has a primarily acquired (oligogenic) disease (**Figure 15.1**).[18] Most recently, based on data from a registry cohort of ARVC patients with implantable cardioverter-defibrillators (ICDs), we found that while all ARVC patients reduce arrhythmic risk by reducing exercise, gene-elusive patients disproportionately benefit (**Figure 15.2**).[19]

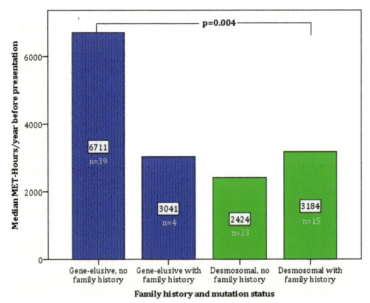

FIGURE 15.1 Association of genotype, family history, and exercise prior to diagnosis among 82 ARVC index patients. Gene-elusive patients with no affected family members per the 2010 TFC on family history had participated in significantly higher-intensity exercise prior to clinical presentation than index patients with desmosomal mutations or gene-elusive patients with affected relatives (P = 0.004), suggesting a disproportionate role of exercise in the etiology of these cases. MET-Hours indicates metabolic equivalent hours. (Reproduced from Sawant et al., *J Am Heart Assoc.* 2014;3(6):e001471.[18])

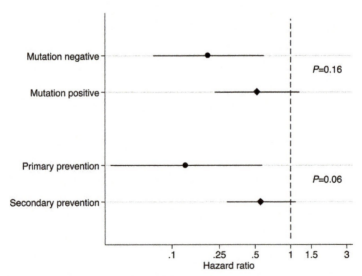

FIGURE 15.2 Impact of exercise reduction after clinical presentation on survival free from appropriate ICD therapy among 129 ARVC patients. Adjusted hazard ratios for ICD therapy for ventricular tachycardia (VT) or ventricular fibrillation (VF) are also presented according to reduction in exercise dose stratified by genotype and primary vs. secondary prevention. Sex, age at presentation (quartiles), primary or secondary prevention, mutation, proband, and annual exercise dose before clinical presentation (quartiles) were adjusted. *P* values for interactions are listed. Overall, greater reduction in exercise dose conferred greater reduction in risk of ventricular arrhythmias (P = 0.01 for trend), but patients without desmosomal mutations and those with primary-prevention ICDs benefited more from exercise reduction (P = 0.16 and P = 0.06 for interaction). (Reproduced from Wang et al., 2018;7(12):10.1161/JAHA.118.008843.[19])

Characterizing Arrhythmic Risk

We also used registry data for a series of studies characterizing clinical factors associated with arrhythmic risk in ARVC. The overarching goal of this work was to inform decision-making for ICD implantation. This included a series of papers on outcomes of patients with ICDs, characterization of patients presenting with SCD, and assessments of a variety of testing modalities and clinical risk factors for predicting incident VAs. Most recently, we characterized predictors of appropriate therapy, outcomes, and complications in 312 definite ARVC patients enrolled in our registry with ICDs and tested utility of a consensus-based risk stratification algorithm for ICD implantation in this population.[20,21] We found that over a mean 8.8 years of follow-up 60% had appropriate therapy and 19% had an appropriate intervention for a rapid VA (VF/flutter, cycle length ≤ 240 ms).[20] As shown in **Figure 15.3**, premature ventricular complexes (PVC) ≥ 1000/24 hours, syncope, age ≤ 30 years at presentation, and male sex were associated with worse survival free from a rapid event in follow-up. Only younger age at presentation (HR: 3.14; 95% CI, 1.32–7.48; $P = 0.010$) and high PVC burden (HR: 4.43; 95% CI, 1.35–14.57; $P < 0.014$) remained independent predictors in multivariable analysis. Notably, a history of sustained VT at presentation, although a predictor of all ICD therapies, was not a significant predictor of experiencing a rapid VA (Panel E).

Using Infrastructure for a Successful National Collaboration: The Dutch Experience

History of the Registry

The Netherlands ACM Registry was established in 2004 under the umbrella of the Interuniversity Cardiology Institute of the Netherlands (now Netherlands Heart Institute). At the time of its inception, the primary aim of this registry was to facilitate research on disease mechanisms, genetics, diagnosis, prognosis, and treatment strategies in ARVC. Over the years, additional objectives were added that include providing education for physicians and patients concerning this disease, for example, through the registry's website (www.acmregistry.nl). In 2018, a first patient and family research seminar was organized together with the patient organization HEARTZ. However, the main focus of the registry is its patient database, which is used to provide new knowledge that may improve management of ARVC patients. Data collection is coordinated by two project leaders (with expertise in the fields of genetics and cardiology, respectively) appointed by the Netherlands Heart Institute.

Structure of the Registry

A detailed description of the Netherlands ACM Registry protocol can be found elsewhere.[22] The Netherlands ACM Registry aims to be inclusive for all arrhythmogenic cardiomyopathies, with ARVC as its most prevalent subtype. In short, the following patients are eligible for inclusion in the Netherlands ACM Registry: (1) definite ARVC patients as confirmed by the diagnostic TFC (after exclusion of alternative diagnoses); (2) their first- and second-degree relatives; and (3) all carriers of pathogenic ARVC-associated mutations, regardless of phenotype. Patients are recruited through all 7 University Medical Centers in the Netherlands permitting near nationwide coverage for enrollment. Phenotypic and outcome data are collected including (but not limited to) ECGs, imaging studies, genetic testing results, ICD interrogations, ventricular/atrial arrhythmias, hospitalizations, and (cardiac) death using standardized data collection instruments. Extensive data quality

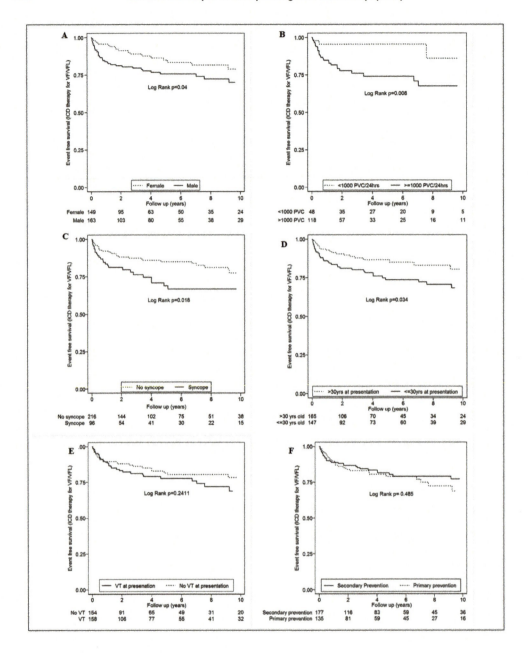

FIGURE 15.3 Cumulative survival from appropriate ICD therapy for rapid VAs (cycle length ≤ 240 ms) among 312 ARVC patients. The panels show outcomes stratified by sex (**A**), PVCs on Holter monitor (**B**), syncope (**C**), age at presentation (**D**), history of VT at presentation (**E**), and primary versus secondary prevention (VT/VF) (**F**). Abbreviations: ICD; implantable cardioverter-defibrillator; PVC, premature ventricular complex; VF/VFL, ventricular fibrillation/flutter; VT/VF, ventricular tachycardia/ventricular fibrillation. (Reproduced from Orgeron et al., *J Am Heart Assoc.* 2017 June 06;6(6):10.1161/ JAHA.117.006242.[20])

control and assurance protocols are in place. As the registry design is observational, management and follow-up intervals remain at the discretion of the participant's own cardiologist. National inclusion of patients is exempt from the Medical Research Involving Human Subjects Act (WMO) as per judgment of the Medical Ethics Committee (METC 18-126/C, Utrecht, The Netherlands). The ACM Registry is registered at the Netherlands Trial Registry, project 7097 (www.trialregister.nl).

Over the last few years, the Netherlands ACM Registry has invested heavily in improvement of data infrastructure. As a result, the registry is currently fully transmitted to an electronic platform (Research Electronic Data Capture [REDCap], Vanderbilt University, Nashville, TN) (**Figure 15.4**). This includes raw data such as ECG images and de-identified cardiac imaging for validation purposes and retrospective collection of newly identified parameters. The REDCap platform has several advantages: Data collection is user-friendly and safe; the system offers the possibility to record all data access, entries, and changes in an audit

trail; and diagnostic criteria for ARVC, dilated cardiomyopathy, and noncompaction cardiomyopathy are automatically calculated by a built-in algorithm that minimizes risk of error. Real-time information on the available data is accessible at https://www.durrercenter.nl/e-detect/. As a result, the Netherlands ACM Registry platform is now up to date with the highest technological standards of data collection, security, privacy, and data-sharing. A modified version has now also been implemented by the Johns Hopkins ARVD/C Program.

Research Foci and Successes

"Traditional" research focuses of the Netherlands ACM Registry over the years have been:

1. **Genetics and genotype/phenotype correlation studies:** We published the ARVC genetic variants database (https://molgenis136.gcc.rug.nl/) and have been involved in discovery of new ARVC-associated genes and studied genotype–phenotype correlations in ARVC.

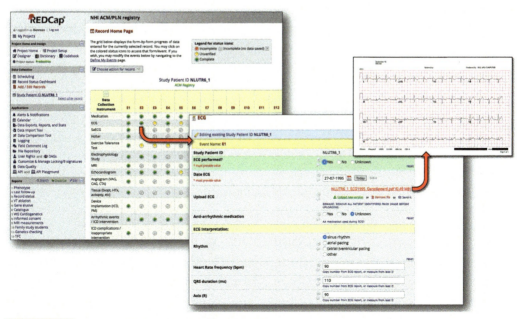

FIGURE 15.4 Schematic of the Netherlands ACM Registry REDCap platform.

2. **Imaging**: We focused on advanced echocardiographic deformation imaging and novel cardiac magnetic resonance (CMR) techniques to improve ARVC diagnosis.
3. **Early detection and family screening**: We described the early ARVC phenotype and determined family screening protocols.

Several of these efforts have been in collaboration with other ARVC registries, so as to increase power for our studies.

Advanced Imaging Studies to Improve Early Disease Detection

Over the years, the Netherlands ACM Registry has built a track record on advanced imaging (echocardiographic deformation imaging and magnetic resonance imaging [MRI]) in ARVC evaluation. In this context, studies on echocardiographic deformation imaging have consistently shown its diagnostic and prognostic value for ARVC evaluation. Already in 2009, we showed that strain-derived parameters have incremental diagnostic value over conventional echocardiography to detect affected ARVC patients,[23] which was subsequently confirmed in asymptomatic mutation carriers.[24] Moreover, we showed that echocardiographic deformation imaging predicts disease development and arrhythmic occurrence in ARVC-associated mutation carriers, suggesting a possible role in early disease detection and risk stratification.[25–27] In addition, several contributions using novel MRI techniques have shown the utility of this technique for ARVC evaluation. Specifically, we showed that MRI-based feature tracking reveals abnormal strain in ARVC-associated mutation carriers prior to overt disease expression[28] and that T1 mapping enables the detection of diffuse fibrosis in ARVC patients.[29]

Risk Assessment and Family Screening

With a small country and short distances between cities, the Netherlands ACM Registry has traditionally included a large proportion of family members: More than 2 in 3 registry participants are relatives. Hence, ARVC family screening has always been of interest to the Netherlands ARVC Registry. Shortly after inception of our registry, we described that genetic testing predicts outcome of ARVC screening in 302 relatives from 93 families,[30] and further family screening studies were performed by one of us (ASJMtR) in collaboration with the Johns Hopkins ARVD/C Program, as described below. Over the years, we also recognized the need for appropriate arrhythmic risk stratification regimens. A comprehensive review and meta-analysis revealed the limitations of prior work[2]: variable definitions and nonuniform study populations, once more highlighting the importance of (international) collaboration. Although the results of this study provided us with an overview of the evidence of single risk factors, additional research studies were needed to translate this to the real-world clinical setting in which patients frequently have multiple risk factors.

Johns Hopkins and Netherlands Registry Integration

In a 2006 *Circulation* issue, the Johns Hopkins and Netherlands ARVC registries independently published manuscripts describing *PKP2* mutations as a major determinant of familial ARVC.[9,31] These manuscripts revealed a remarkably similar presentation, clinical phenotype, and natural history among North American and Dutch ARVC patients, and indeed each reported an identical prevalence (43%) of *PKP2* mutations. These similarities did not go unnoticed, and the 2 program leaders at the time, Hugh Calkins and Richard Hauer, began to discuss collaboration and arranged the first of many exchanges of student researchers. A publication comprehensively characterizing desmosomal variants among Johns Hopkins Registry enrollees was the result,[32] and Dr. Hauer came to Baltimore as the featured guest speaker at the Johns Hopkins Family ARVC seminar to share the experiences of the Netherlands ARVC program. This combination of rigorous science and personal connection strengthened by exchange of personnel and regular in-person meetings has been the recipe for our successful collaboration ever since.

The first large collaborative project of the Netherlands and Johns Hopkins registries was to define genotype–phenotype relationships. As this necessitated stratification of the population for analysis, and both the Netherlands and Johns Hopkins ARVC registries had an overwhelming preponderance of *PKP2* variants, neither program could tackle this question alone. This project first required consensus on definitions for predictor variables and outcomes. A lengthy standard operating procedure defining variables was jointly developed and data abstraction piloted by each registry. Analyses were performed to confirm similar baseline characteristics and appropriateness of merging the cohorts. Planning also required a common definition for what constituted a pathogenic variant (mutation). We developed a consensus-based approach with all variants first adjudicated independently by Dutch and U.S. genetics teams with conflicts and uncertainty resolved in a series of conference calls. The work done to develop common definitions of predictors and outcomes of interest as well as a common approach to defining pathogenicity of variants provided a resource used not only in this initial project but also for research studies that followed and served as the basis of our aligned REDCap databases.

Building on this dataset, common definitions for outcomes and predictors, and similar approach to genotyping and variant adjudica-tion a series of collaborative projects followed. The datasets were expanded to include detailed CMR analyses, echocardiographic findings, pregnancy outcomes, and extended sequencing data. Over the years, the combined Johns Hopkins–Netherlands dataset led to 23 research manuscripts to date added to the literature. We highlight 3 areas of joint successes that would have been impossible without a collaborative approach next.

Joint Successes

Genotype/Phenotype Relationships

This first collaborative effort resulted in a cohort of 1001 genotyped ARVC patients and family members that we used to define genotype–phenotype relationships and generate new insights into natural history. We found that, broadly, gene-positive and gene-elusive probands have a similar disease course although gene-positive cases present at a younger age on average. In contrast, as shown in **Figure 15.5**, family genotype strongly predicts likelihood a relative will develop sustained VT, require a transplant or die from ARVC.[33] In our cohort there were no ARVC-related deaths, and only 2 patients (1%) with sustained VAs recorded among 152 first-degree relatives of gene-elusive patients. We also found genotype predicts extent of left ventricular (LV) involvement and likelihood of heart failure.[34] LV dysfunction was present in more than half of probands with *PLN* and *DSP* variants but only 15% of those with *PKP2* and 30% of *DSG2* carriers with a similar pattern, but lower prevalence, in family members. We also found that among gene-positive cases, SCD/arrest presentation occurred disproportionately among the youngest individuals and that those with *DSP* variants were particularly likely to have such a presentation. Finally, the small cohort of patients with multiple mutations had a significantly worse clinical course.

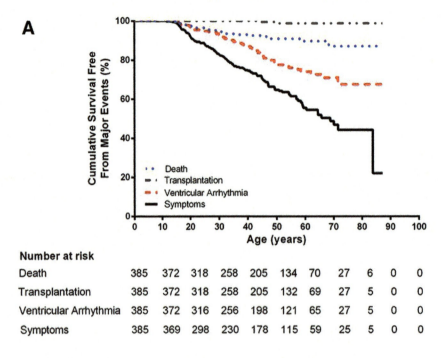

Number at risk

Death	385	372	318	258	205	134	70	27	6	0	0
Transplantation	385	372	318	258	205	132	69	27	5	0	0
Ventricular Arrhythmia	385	372	316	256	198	121	65	27	5	0	0
Symptoms	385	369	298	230	178	115	59	25	5	0	0

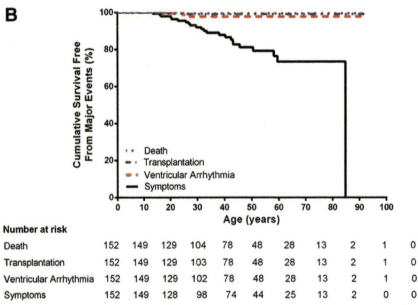

Number at risk

Death	152	149	129	104	78	48	28	13	2	1	0
Transplantation	152	149	129	103	78	48	28	13	2	1	0
Ventricular Arrhythmia	152	149	129	102	78	48	28	13	2	1	0
Symptoms	152	149	128	98	74	44	25	13	2	0	0

FIGURE 15.5 Association of genotype with outcomes of 537 at-risk relatives is presented. The panels show survival free from any ARVC–related symptoms (**black**), sustained VAs (**red**), cardiac death (**blue**), and cardiac transplantation (**grey**) in 385 gene-positive family members of gene-positive index cases (**A**) and 152 first-degree relatives of gene-elusive index cases (**B**). Family members of gene-elusive index cases had significantly better outcomes with only 2 sustained VAs ($P < 0.001$) and no deaths. (Reproduced from Groeneweg et al., *Circ Cardiovasc Genet.* 2015;8(3):437–446.[33])

Toward Evidence-Based Family Screening Approaches

Our next stage of collaboration was facilitated by the PhD work conducted jointly in Baltimore and Utrecht by one of us (ASJtR), which focused in part on the challenging question of family screening. In these studies, we established that evidence of electrical abnormalities precedes or occurs simultaneously with structural disease,[35,36] an insight that helps plan strategies for family screening. We next assembled a joint cohort of 274 first-degree relatives with full cardiovascular evaluations and follow-up data.[37] Approximately one-third (n = 96, 35%) developed definite ARVC. In these well-characterized relatives, independent predictors of diagnosis included age, symptoms, genotype, and being a sibling rather than a parent or child. While being a sibling was a predictor of ARVC diagnosis, neither relatedness to the proband nor malignant family history was significantly associated with arrhythmic events. Meeting TFC independent of family history criteria had higher prognostic value for arrhythmic events than conventional 2010 TFC. These studies were very informative for our clinical practices and continue to inform our family screening approaches.

Genetic Architecture of ARVC

Most recently we have leveraged our collaboration to more thoroughly define the genetic architecture of ARVC. This research area was strengthened by the sabbatical of one of us (CAJ) in the Netherlands with J. Peter van Tintelen, MD, PhD. We jointly re-adjudicated the pathogenicity of all variants in the registries. An analysis of 501 genotyped ARVC probands and their families (including a cohort from Germany) revealed that pathogenic desmosomal ARVC variants are seldom de novo, infrequently unique,

and based on haplotype likely derived from ancient founders (**Figure 15.6**).[36] This insight has important implications for genetic testing strategy and also the penetrance of desmosomal variants in the general population. Currently members of our programs are leading the international ARVC Gene Curation Expert Panel to reexamine evidence for gene–disease associations in ARVC under the auspices of ClinGen (https://clinicalgenome.org/affiliation/40003/).[39]

Predicting Arrhythmic Risk

We next sought to return to our early questions about arrhythmia risk prediction with the goal of deriving a model to estimate individualized risk of incident arrhythmias. To prepare for this study, the Netherlands and Johns Hopkins programs each led a preparatory analysis. The Dutch team led an extensive systematic review and meta-analysis of all clinical parameters associated with an increased risk of VAs.[2] The Johns Hopkins team tested an existing risk-stratification algorithm proposed by a panel of international experts and found opportunities for improvement.[21]

In light of these results, it was clear that the crucial question of risk stratification in ARVC had to be addressed in a well-powered study, and that undertaking this task would require an unparalleled collaboration extending beyond our two groups. We were lucky that the connection could be established very naturally when key players of the Zurich and of the Nordic registry, Dr. Firat Duru and Dr. Pyotr Platonov, both visited Baltimore for invited lectures and through the connections of the first author (JCT) with her home institutions the Montreal Heart Institute and the Canadian ARVC Registry. This unparalleled group effort led to the creation of the largest cohort of definite ARVC patients without a prior history of sustained arrhythmic events (primary prevention) with a total of 528 patients (**Figure 15.7**).

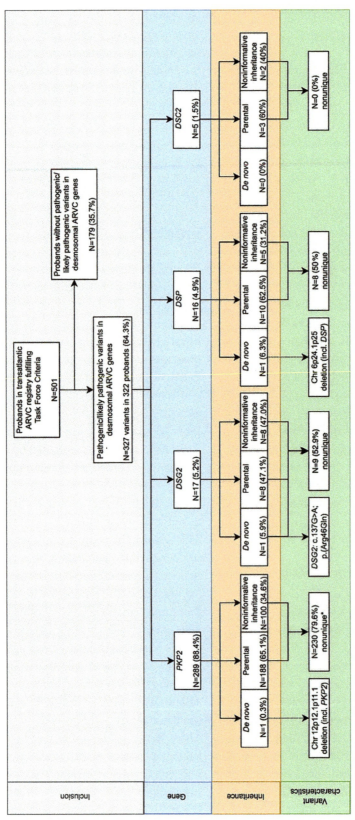

FIGURE 15.6 Inheritance of desmosomal variants is presented. Inheritance of desmosomal variants identified among 501 probands with ARVC from the Johns Hopkins Registry, the Netherlands Registry, and a German center is shown. Variants were disproportionately found in *PKP2*, were rarely de novo, and were characterized by recurrent variants with shared haplotypes across registries. Chr indicates chromosome. *230 probands carried 26 different nonunique variants in *PKP2*. For 24 nonunique variants, haplotype analysis has been performed in 183 families using 260 samples. (Reproduced from van Lint et al., *Circ Genom Precis Med.* 2019;12(8):e002467.[38])

This fruitful collaboration allowed the creation of an adequate risk prediction model for sustained VA (Figure 15.7) incorporating clinical predictors identified from prior literature including the above-mentioned meta-analysis.[40] The algorithm includes age, sex, history of recent syncope, history of nonsustained VT, RV ejection fraction, PVCs per 24 hours, and extent of T-wave inversions on ECG. The online risk calculator associated with its publication in *European Heart Journal* in 2019 has now received more than 9735 visits illustrating its uptake in clinical practice (www.ARVCrisk .com). The performance of the risk calculator was recently validated in both a small external Italian cohort and a cohort of athletic ARVC patients.[41,42]

Toward the Future

It is clear that the ARVC community is a close community with strong interinstitutional communication and collaboration. We all strive to address important knowledge gaps in the field, which include (but are not limited to (1) identification of the genetic (e.g., additional genes) and environmental (e.g., exercise) factors that modify disease expression and outcomes; (2) better definition of pathogenicity of genes associated with ARVC; (3) more insights into the population incidence and prevalence of ARVC; (4) further refinement in personalized risk prediction and management for both arrhythmia and heart failure risks; and (5) determination of disease-specific

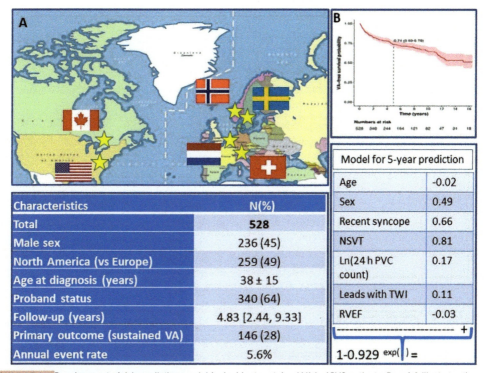

FIGURE 15.7 Development of risk prediction model for incident sustained VA in ARVC patients. **Panel A** illustrates the different countries involved, which includes Canada, United States, Norway, Sweden, the Netherlands, and Switzerland. **Panel B** illustrates the cumulative survival free from any sustained VA along with the 95% confidence intervals (**shaded area**). The **dotted line** represents the cumulative 5-year survival. Abbreviations: NSVT, nonsustained VT; PVC, premature ventricular complexes; RVEF, right ventricular ejection fraction; TWI, T-wave inversion. (Figure made based on published data from Cadrin-Tourigny et al., *Expert Rev Cardiovasc Ther.* 2019 August 21:1–7.[40])

pathogenic pathways and potential therapeutic targets. A comprehensive overview of research priorities described by experts in the field has been recently published.[43]

To address these research priorities, we believe that an expansion of already existing collaborations can lead to further advances in the field. For example, the REDCap infrastructure that is already adopted by the Johns Hopkins and Netherlands ARVC/ACM registries provides a unique opportunity to align data on a uniform and secure data platform and ultimately facilitate data sharing. Building translational collaborations between preclinical and clinical research programs may provide important insights on the pathophysiology of disease and lead to potential therapeutic targets. We very much welcome new collaborations in hopes that it benefits our joint mission: to further improve our understanding of this disease and to provide excellent care for our patients.

As a postscript, this chapter has been written during the COVID-19 outbreak with the authors socially distanced in 3 nations across 2 continents. Never has the world seemed so small and international collaboration and friendship felt so important.

References

1. Marcus FI, Fontaine GH, Guiraudon G, Frank R, Laurenceau JL, Malergue C, et al. Right ventricular dysplasia: A report of 24 adult cases. *Circulation*. 1982;65(2):384–398.
2. Bosman LP, Sammani A, James CA, Cadrin-Tourigny J, Calkins H, van Tintelen JP, et al. Predicting arrhythmic risk in arrhythmogenic right ventricular cardiomyopathy: A systematic review and meta-analysis. *Heart Rhythm*. 2018;15(7):1097–1107.
3. James CA, Calkins H. Arrhythmogenic right ventricular cardiomyopathy: Progress toward personalized management. *Annu Rev Med*. 2019;70:1–18.
4. James CA, Syrris P, van Tintelen JP, Calkins H. The role of genetics in cardiovascular disease: Arrhythmogenic cardiomyopathy. *Eur Heart J*. 2020;41(14):1393–1400.
5. Gupta R, Tichnell C, Murray B, et al. Comparison of features of fatal versus nonfatal cardiac arrest in patients with arrhythmogenic right ventricular dysplasia/cardiomyopathy. *Am J Cardiol*. 2017;120(1):111–117.
6. Marcus FI, McKenna WJ, Sherrill D, et al. Diagnosis of arrhythmogenic right ventricular cardiomyopathy/dysplasia: Proposed modification of the Task Force Criteria. *Eur Heart J*. 2010;31(7):806–814.
7. Chelko SP, James C, Tichnell C, Murray B. The Johns Hopkins ARVC International Symposium. *Eur Heart J*. 2019;40(29):2387–2389.
8. Dalal D, Nasir K, Bomma C, et al. Arrhythmogenic right ventricular dysplasia: A United States experience. *Circulation*. 2005;112(25):3823–3832.
9. Dalal D, Molin LH, Piccini J, Tichnell C, James C, Bomma C, et al. Clinical features of arrhythmogenic right ventricular dysplasia/cardiomyopathy associated with mutations in plakophilin-2. *Circulation*. 2006;113(13):1641–1649.
10. Dalal D, James C, Devanagondi R, Tichnell C, Tucker A, Prakasa K, et al. Penetrance of mutations in plakophilin-2 among families with arrhythmogenic right ventricular dysplasia/cardiomyopathy. *J Am Coll Cardiol*. 2006;48(7):1416–1424.
11. Awad MM, Dalal D, Cho E, Amat-Alarcon N, James C, Tichnell C, et al. DSG2 mutations contribute to arrhythmogenic right ventricular dysplasia/cardiomyopathy. *Am J Hum Genet*. 2006;79(1):136–142.
12. Bomma C, Dalal D, Tandri H, Prakasa K, Nasir K, Roguin A, et al. Evolving role of multidetector computed tomography in evaluation of arrhythmogenic right ventricular dysplasia/cardiomyopathy. *Am J Cardiol*. 2007;100(1):99–105.
13. Tops LF, Prakasa K, Tandri H, Dalal D, Jain R, Dimaano VL, et al. Prevalence and pathophysiologic attributes of ventricular dyssyn-

chrony in arrhythmogenic right ventricular dysplasia/cardiomyopathy. *J Am Coll Cardiol.* 2009;54(5):445–451.

14. Tandri H, Bluemke DA, Ferrari VA, et al. Findings on magnetic resonance imaging of idiopathic right ventricular outflow tachycardia. *Am J Cardiol.* 2004;94(11):1441–1445.

15. Bomma C, Dalal D, Tandri H, et al. Regional differences in systolic and diastolic function in arrhythmogenic right ventricular dysplasia/cardiomyopathy using magnetic resonance imaging. *Am J Cardiol.* 2005;95(12):1507–1511.

16. James CA, Bhonsale A, Tichnell C, et al. Exercise increases age-related penetrance and arrhythmic risk in arrhythmogenic right ventricular dysplasia/cardiomyopathy-associated desmosomal mutation carriers. *J Am Coll Cardiol.* 2013;62(14):1290–1297.

17. Sawant AC, te Riele AS, Tichnell C, et al. Safety of American Heart Association-recommended minimum exercise for desmosomal mutation carriers. *Heart Rhythm.* 2016;13(1):199–207.

18. Sawant AC, Bhonsale A, te Riele AS, et al. Exercise has a disproportionate role in the pathogenesis of arrhythmogenic right ventricular dysplasia/cardiomyopathy in patients without desmosomal mutations. *J Am Heart Assoc.* 2014;3(6):e001471.

19. Wang W, Orgeron G, Tichnell C, et al. Impact of exercise restriction on arrhythmic risk among patients with arrhythmogenic right ventricular cardiomyopathy. *J Am Heart Assoc.* 2018;7(12):10.1161/JAHA.118.008843.

20. Orgeron GM, James CA, te Riele A, et al. Implantable cardioverter-defibrillator therapy in arrhythmogenic right ventricular dysplasia/cardiomyopathy: Predictors of appropriate therapy, outcomes, and complications. *J Am Heart Assoc.* 2017;6(6):10.1161/JAHA.117.006242.

21. Orgeron GM, te Riele A, Tichnell C, et al. Performance of the 2015 International Task Force Consensus Statement risk stratification algorithm for implantable cardioverter-defibrillator placement in arrhythmogenic right ventricular dysplasia/cardiomyopathy. *Circ Arrhythmia Electrophysiol.* 2018;11(2):e005593.

22. Bosman LP, Verstraelen TE, van Lint FHM, et al. The Netherlands Arrhythmogenic Cardiomyopathy Registry: Design and status update. *Neth Heart J.* 2019;27:480–486.

23. Teske AJ, Cox MG, De Boeck BW, Doevendans PA, Hauer RN, Cramer MJ. Echocardiographic tissue deformation imaging quantifies abnormal regional right ventricular function in arrhythmogenic right ventricular dysplasia/cardiomyopathy. *J Am Soc Echocardiogr.* 2009;22(8):920–927.

24. Teske AJ, Cox MG, te Riele AS, et al. Early detection of regional functional abnormalities in asymptomatic ARVD/C gene carriers. *J Am Soc Echocardiogr.* 2012;25(9):997–1006.

25. Mast TP, Taha K, Cramer MJ, et al. The prognostic value of right ventricular deformation imaging in early arrhythmogenic right ventricular cardiomyopathy. *JACC Cardiovasc Imaging.* 2018; 2(3):446–455.

26. Mast TP, Teske AJ, Walmsley J, et al. Right ventricular imaging and computer simulation for electromechanical substrate characterization in arrhythmogenic right ventricular cardiomyopathy. *J Am Coll Cardiol.* 2016;68(20):2185–2197.

27. Mast TP, Teske AJ, te Riele AS, et al. Prolonged electromechanical interval unmasks arrhythmogenic right ventricular dysplasia/cardiomyopathy in the subclinical stage. *J Cardiovasc Electrophysiol.* 2016;27(3):303–314.

28. Bourfiss M, Vigneault DM, Aliyari Ghasebeh M, et al. Feature tracking CMR reveals abnormal strain in preclinical arrhythmogenic right ventricular dysplasia/ cardiomyopathy: A multisoftware feasibility and clinical implementation study. *J Cardiovasc Magn Reson.* 2017;19(1):66–64.

29. Bourfiss M, Prakken NHJ, van der Heijden JF, et al. Diagnostic value of native T1 mapping in arrhythmogenic right ventricular cardiomyopathy. *JACC Cardiovasc Imaging.* 2019;12(8 Pt 1):1580–1582.

30. Cox MG, van der Zwaag PA, van der Werf C, et al. Arrhythmogenic right ventricular dysplasia/cardiomyopathy: Pathogenic desmosome mutations in index-patients predict outcome of family screening: Dutch arrhythmogenic

right ventricular dysplasia/cardiomyopathy genotype-phenotype follow-up study. *Circulation.* 2011;123(23):2690–2700.

31. van Tintelen JP, Entius MM, Bhuiyan ZA, et al. Plakophilin-2 mutations are the major determinant of familial arrhythmogenic right ventricular dysplasia/cardiomyopathy. *Circulation.* 2006;113(13):1650–1658.

32. den Haan AD, Tan BY, Zikusoka MN, et al. Comprehensive desmosome mutation analysis in north americans with arrhythmogenic right ventricular dysplasia/cardiomyopathy. *Circ Cardiovasc Genet.* 2009;2(5):428–435.

33. Groeneweg JA, Bhonsale A, James CA, et al. Clinical presentation, long-term follow-up, and outcomes of 1001 arrhythmogenic right ventricular dysplasia/cardiomyopathy patients and family members. *Circ Cardiovasc Genet.* 2015;8(3):437–446.

34. Bhonsale A, Groeneweg JA, James CA, et al. Impact of genotype on clinical course in arrhythmogenic right ventricular dysplasia/cardiomyopathy-associated mutation carriers. *Eur Heart J.* 2015;36(14):847–855.

35. te Riele AS, Bhonsale A, James CA, et al. Incremental value of cardiac magnetic resonance imaging in arrhythmic risk stratification of arrhythmogenic right ventricular dysplasia/cardiomyopathy-associated desmosomal mutation carriers. *J Am Coll Cardiol.* 2013;62(19):1761–1769.

36. te Riele AS, James CA, Rastegar N, et al. Yield of serial evaluation in at-risk family members of patients with ARVD/C. *J Am Coll Cardiol.* 2014;64(3):293–301.

37. te Riele AS, James CA, Groeneweg JA, et al. Approach to family screening in arrhythmogenic right ventricular dysplasia/cardiomyopathy. *Eur Heart J.* 2016;37(9):755–763.

38. van Lint FHM, Murray B, Tichnell C, et al. Arrhythmogenic right ventricular cardiomyopathy-associated desmosomal variants are rarely de novo. *Circ Genom Precis Med.* 2019;12(8):e002467.

39. Rehm HL, Berg JS, Brooks LD, et al. ClinGen—the clinical genome resource. *N Engl J Med.* 2015;372(23):2235–2242.

40. Cadrin-Tourigny J, Bosman LP, Tadros R, et al. Risk stratification for ventricular arrhythmias and sudden cardiac death in arrhythmogenic right ventricular cardiomyopathy: An update. *Expert Rev Cardiovasc Ther.* 2019 August 21:1–7.

41. Casella M, Gasperetti A, Gaetano F, et al. Long-term follow-up analysis of a highly characterized arrhythmogenic cardiomyopathy cohort with classical and non-classical phenotypes-a real-world assessment of a novel prediction model: Does the subtype really matter? *Europace.* 2020;22(5):797–805.

42. Gasperetti A, Russo AD, Busana M, et al. Novel risk calculator performance in athletes with arrhythmogenic right ventricular cardiomyopathy. *Heart Rhythm.* 2020;17(8):1251–1259.

43. Elliott PM, Anastasakis A, Asimaki A, et al. Definition and treatment of arrhythmogenic cardiomyopathy: An updated expert panel report. *Eur J Heart Fail.* 2019;21(8):955–964.

16

The Role of Protein Redistribution in the Diagnosis of Arrhythmogenic Cardiomyopathy: A Translational Perspective

Carlos Bueno-Beti, PhD; Angeliki Asimaki, PhD

Introduction

The Disease

Classically, we think of arrhythmogenic cardiomyopathy (ACM) as a disease in which the myocardium is replaced by fat and fibrous tissue. While this change may become especially prominent as the disease progresses, it is not uncommon for patients to manifest life-threatening arrhythmias with minimal or no histological abnormalities.[1] It is therefore of pivotal importance to understand the molecular mechanisms of disease pathogenesis in order to diagnose it early and prevent sudden cardiac death (SCD).

Approximately 50% of ACM patients bear one or more mutations in genes encoding for desmosomal proteins.[2] Desmosomes are intercellular adhesion junctions, which in cardiac myocytes reside within the intercalated disk (ID). They consist of members of the cadherin family, namely desmoglein-2 (Dsg2) and desmocollin-2 (Dsc2), as well as members of the plakin and armadillo families, namely plakoglobin (JUP), plakophilin-2 (PKP2), and desmoplakin (DSP), which link the cadherins to the intermediate filaments of the cytoskeleton providing the myocardium with mechanical strength.[3] Some desmosomal proteins, in particular JUP, have dual roles as structural proteins in cell–cell adhesion junctions and as nuclear signaling molecules, suggesting that the pathogenesis of ACM is related to a combination of altered cellular biomechanical behavior and altered signaling.[4]

Protein Remodeling in the ACM Myocardium

Plakoglobin

To gain insights into the mechanisms through which desmosomal gene mutations cause ACM, Dr. Saffitz's group analyzed myocardial samples obtained at autopsy or through endomyocardial biopsy (EMB) from ACM patients. The first question they aimed to answer was whether the mutant desmosomal protein is expressed, and if so, whether it localizes at the cell–cell junctions.[5] Kaplan et al. initially examined myocardium from patients with Naxos disease, a rare, recessive, syndromic form of the disease associated with hair and skin abnormalities related to an underlying mutation in *JUP* (2157del2).[6,7] Immunohistochemical studies showed that the mutant *JUP* fails to reach the IDs, while Western blot studies showed that the truncated protein is clearly expressed.[7] Kaplan et al. next examined myocardial samples from a patient with Carvajal syndrome, another recessive syndromic form of the disease with an underlying mutation in *DSP*.[8,9] This analysis showed that in Carvajal syndrome, not only did the mutant protein, DSP, fail to localize at the IDs, but so did its binding partner, JUP. This observation provided the first evidence that a mutation in a single protein may perturb the subcellular distribution of another protein that is not itself genetically altered.[9]

We next studied myocardium from large numbers of patients with clinically and/or pathologically documented ACM. We found that single-gene mutations cause variable patterns of altered localization of desmosomal proteins even when the mutation affects only a single allele. This suggested that the mutant protein alters binding interactions within the ID, causing further proteins to redistribute from junctional to cytosolic compartments and potentially change nuclear signaling and gene expression patterns. We also found that in the vast majority of ACM cases, immunoreactive signal for JUP was virtually absent from the IDs (**Figure 16.1**). This relocalization appeared to be specific among the cardiomyopathies as we did not observe a similar shift in cases of hypertrophic cardiomyopathy (HCM), dilated cardiomyopathy (DCM), or ischemic cardiomyopathy.[10]

Although ACM is traditionally regarded as "a disease of the desmosome," several recent studies have now shown that nondesmosomal gene mutations may also underlie forms of the disease. Phospholamban (PLN) is a regulator of the sarcoplasmic reticulum

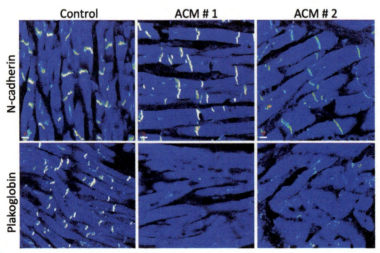

FIGURE 16.1 Plakoglobin shifts from junctional to intracellular pools in ACM. Representative confocal immunofluorescence images showing depressed signal for plakoglobin at the cardiac intercalated disks in myocardium from 2 patients with ACM compared to a healthy control. Signal for N-cadherin, used as a tissue quality marker, was strong in both ACM cases and indistinguishable from controls.

Ca^{2+} (SERCA2a) pump in cardiac muscle and thus important for maintaining Ca^{2+} homeostasis. The same mutation in *PLN* (R14del) has been shown to underlie cases of both ACM and DCM. Interestingly, we showed that JUP fails to reach the IDs in R14del *PLN* mutation-carriers diagnosed with ACM while it showed control distribution in bearers of the exact same mutation manifesting with a DCM phenotype (**Figure 16.2**).[11] This finding suggested that the inability of JUP to localize at the IDs correlates with the disease phenotype as opposed to the genotype of the patient.

Connexin43

An extensive literature exists on the dependence of cell–cell coupling at gap junctions on the formation and maintenance of mechanical junctions.[12] Kaplan et al. first showed gap junction remodeling in Naxos disease and Carvajal syndrome.[7,9] Subsequently, however, we showed that connexin43 (Cx43) signal is significantly depressed at the IDs in the vast majority of ACM forms regardless of the underlying mutation.[10] Gap junction remodeling is not specific to ACM and has been reported in several cases of ischemic and nonischemic heart disease. There is, however, one fundamental difference: In other cardiomyopathies, such reduction in Cx43 signal is more apparent in advanced disease, in which there has been considerable structural remodeling of the heart. In contrast, gap junction remodeling in patients with ACM occurs diffusely in regions of the heart that show no apparent structural or functional alterations. This is a potentially important distinction adding to the growing body of literature supporting that gap junction remodeling is a primary driving force of conduction abnormalities and arrhythmogenesis in ACM.

Nav1.5

Silencing of PKP2 *in vitro* leads to decreased sodium current (I_{Na}).[13] Additionally, PKP2-haploinsufficient mice show a significant I_{Na} deficiency.[14] Given the close proximity and the numerous binding interactions between members of ion channels, mechanical, and electrical junctions within the ID,[15] it was not surprising that signal for Nav1.5, the major protein subunit of the cardiac sodium

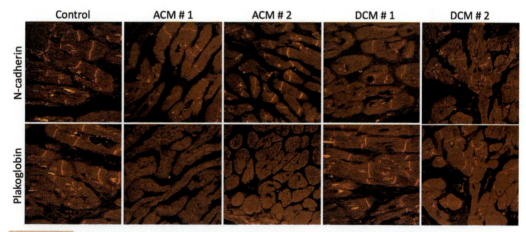

FIGURE 16.2 Loss of junctional plakoglobin signal in *PLN* R14del carriers with an ACM but not a DCM phenotype. Representative confocal immunofluorescence images of myocardium from 2 patients diagnosed with ACM and 2 patients diagnosed with DCM, all carrying the *PLN* R14del mutation, compared to a control sample. Immunoreactive signal for plakoglobin was depressed in the ACM but not the DCM samples.[11]

channel, was also significantly depressed at the cardiac IDs in a large number of ACM patient samples analyzed.[16]

Delmar's group was the first to show reduced densities of the cardiac I_{Na} current in experimental models of ACM.[13,14] Subsequently, Dr. Kleber confirmed this finding in further models of the disease and also showed for the first time a significant reduction in the inward rectifying potassium current, I_{K1}, in the presence of ACM-causing mutations.[17] These alterations, combined with reduced gap junctional coupling, could contribute to the highly arrhythmogenic phenotype of the disease. Only limited characterization of cellular electrophysiology has been performed in patients with ACM; this involves analysis of cardiac myocytes from patient-derived induced pluripotent stem cells (iPSC-CMs). Such cells from an ACM patient bearing a mutation in *PKP2* showed reduced I_{Na}[18] and abnormal Ca^{2+} dynamics.[19] These observations raise the possibility that defective localization of ion channel proteins could contribute to reduced I_{Na} and I_{K1} densities in ACM. In this regard, the PDZ domain protein synapse-associated protein 97 (SAP97) is known to participate in the trafficking and targeting of Nav1.5 and Kir2.1 (the major protein subunit responsible for the I_{K1} current) to the membrane.[20]

Synapse-Associated Protein 97

To further investigate the role of SAP97 in ACM, we knocked down its expression in normal neonatal rat ventricular myocytes (NRVMs) using short hairpin RNA (shRNA) and examined the distribution of key ID proteins.[17] Knock-down of SAP97 prevented junctional localization of Nav1.5 as reported. However, it also reduced junctional localization of JUP but not of other desmosomal proteins, including PKP2 and DSP. This unexpected observation suggested a central role for SAP97 in the localization of both JUP and

ion channel proteins in the cell membrane. It also suggested a role for abnormal protein trafficking in the pathogenesis of ACM. We next examined the localization of SAP97 in human myocardial samples. In control samples, SAP97 shows sarcomeric distribution with more intense signal localization at the IDs. In myocardium from patients with ACM; however, there is a significant drop of signal in both sarcomeric and ID compartments. In other forms of heart disease examined, including HCM, DCM, ischemia, and cardiac sarcoidosis, signal for SAP97 is absent at the IDs but still present at the sarcomeres. Accordingly, absence of SAP97 signal altogether appeared to be a specific feature of ACM (**Figure 16.3**).[17]

Glycogen Synthase Kinase 3β (GSK3β) and Adenomatous Polyposis Coli (APC)

To gain further insights into disease mechanisms and facilitate high-throughput chemical screening for drug discovery, in collaboration with Dr. MacRae, we created a transgenic zebrafish model of ACM with cardiac-specific expression of *JUP* bearing the *2157del2* mutation. The mutant fish exhibit bradycardia, reduced stroke volume, and reduced cardiac output by only 48 hours post-fertilization. Soon after, they develop cardiomegaly, peripheral edema, and cachexia. They show increased mortality by the time maturity is reached.[17] We used this model to screen a library of bioactive compounds for disease modifiers. One compound, SB216763, prevented the development of bradycardia and contractility defects and significantly increased survival in the mutant fish. It also prevented all disease-associated end points in *in vitro* models of ACM (NRVMs expressing disease-causing mutations as well as patient-derived iPSC-CMs).[17] More importantly, it prevented both clinical and subcellular disease features in 2 different murine models of

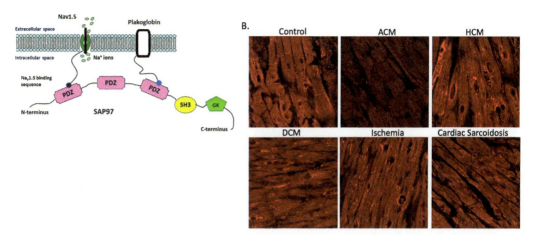

FIGURE 16.3   Remodeling of SAP97 localization in ACM. **Panel A:** Schematic representation of SAP97 binding both Nav1.5 and plakoglobin targeting them to the cell membrane. **Panel B:** Representative images showing loss of SAP97 signal in myocardium from a patient with ACM compared to a healthy control. SAP97 is lost from the junctions but retained at the sarcomeres in cases of HCM, DCM, ischemia, and cardiac sarcoidosis.[17]

ACM: A transgenic mouse with cardiac specific expression of *JUP* bearing the *2157del2* mutation and a homozygous knock-in of mutant *Dsg2*.[21] SB216763 has been annotated as a specific inhibitor of glycogen synthase kinase 3β (GSK3β). Although this small molecule can mitigate both the arrhythmia and myocardial injury phenotypes of ACM in a wide range of experimental models, long-term inhibition of GSK3β in patients could have unacceptable adverse consequences, including increased risk of developing cancer.[22] Despite it being inappropriate for patient use, the identification of SB216763 did focus our attention on the key role GSK3β appears to be playing in the pathogenesis of ACM.

Accordingly, we next investigated the localization of this enzyme in the human heart. Under basal conditions, GSK3β resides in the cytoplasm, where it forms a complex with adenomatous polyposis coli (APC), casein kinase II (CKII), and an axin known as the degradation complex. Its role is to phosphorylate target proteins, earmarking them for ubiquitination and proteasomal degradation. The most heavily researched protein in which turnover is regulated through this complex is β-catenin, a protein closely related to JUP

(**Figure 16.4A**).[23,24] In healthy human myocardium, GSK3β and its binding partner APC show a diffuse cytosolic localization. In sharp contrast, both proteins localize at the IDs in myocardium from patients with ACM. This "reverse remodeling of the ID" was unique to ACM, as we did not observe it in any other form of heart disease we examined, including HCM, DCM, and ischemia (Figure 16.4B).[21]

The Molecular Signature of ACM

Not all protein redistributions hitherto reviewed are specific to ACM, but their combination is shown to constitute a rather robust molecular signature for the classical form of the disease. Immunohistochemical analysis of the vast majority of predominantly right ventricular forms of ACM cases examined has shown a shift of JUP, Cx43, Nav1.5, and SAP97 from junctional to intracellular pools while GSK3β and APC translocate from the cytosol to the cell–cell junctions (**Figure 16.5**). To date, the combination of these markers has aided diagnosis of several equivocal cases. It is, however, significantly limited by the implicit need for a myocardial sample.

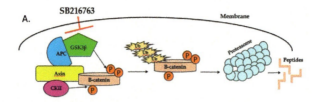

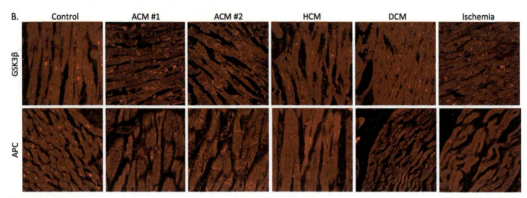

FIGURE 16.4   Redistribution of the degradation complex in ACM. **Panel A:** Schematic diagram of the degradation complex. **Panel B:** Representative confocal images showing cytosolic localization of GSK3β and APC in control myocardium and concentration of signal at the intercalated disks in myocardium from patients with ACM but not in other cardiomyopathies.[21]

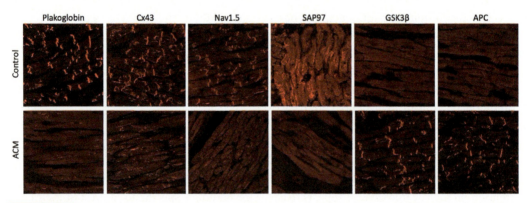

FIGURE 16.5   The molecular signature of ACM. Typical localization of plakoglobin, Cx43, Nav1.5, SAP97, GSK3β, and APC in control myocardium versus myocardium from a patient with ACM.

Protein Remodeling in the ACM Buccal Epithelium

Endomyocardial biopsies are difficult and risky to obtain from patients and virtually impossible to obtain from genotype-positive family members who do not show any clinical manifestation of disease but may still be at risk of SCD. A few studies have used iPSC-CMs derived from affected and unaffected carriers of ACM-causing mutations, but this approach is expensive, technically demanding, and very time-consuming.[19,25] To find a surrogate tissue for the heart that we could use to analyze key protein marker localization in probands and carrier family members, we investigated buccal mucosa cells, which can be easily and safely obtained from large numbers of people at a minimal cost.[26]

The buccal epithelium consists of flattened, squamous cells with small central nuclei and clearly identifiable edges. Immunostaining studies showed strong membranous signal for JUP, Cx43, DSP, and PKP1; an isoform of PKP2 is expressed at the upper epithelia. No signal was detected in buccal mucosa cells for PKP2, the isoform expressed in the heart (**Figure 16.6**).[26]

To determine whether the localization of junctional proteins is altered in the buccal epithelium in patients with ACM, we obtained smears from 39 patients with clinically documented disease and a known mutation in a desmosomal gene. This included 25 patients with an autosomal dominant mutation in *PKP2*, 4 patients with a dominant mutation in *Dsg2*, 2 patients with a dominant mutation in *Dsc2*, 2 patients with a dominant mutation in *DSP*, and 6 patients with Naxos disease, homozygous for the 2157del2 mutation in *JUP*. Of

these 39 patients, 87% showed clearly reduced immunoreactive signal for JUP, and 97% of patients showed near absent signal for Cx43 in their buccal smears compared to samples from 40 ethnically and age-matched healthy controls. Those patients bearing a mutation in *Dsc2*, *Dsg2* or *DSP* showed depressed signal for DSP in their buccal mucosa but not for PKP1. Conversely, patients bearing a mutation in *PKP2*, showed depressed signal for PKP1 but not for DSP (**Figure 16.7**).[26] This association becomes more remarkable when one considers that PKP1 and PKP2 are encoded by different genes, located on different chromosomes. PKP2 is expressed in the heart and in basal cells of the epidermis but not in keratinocytes or buccal mucosa cells.[27,28] Whether progenitors of buccal mucosa cells express PKP2 is not known, but these results suggest common regulatory mechanisms between the 2 protein isoforms. Signal for JUP and Cx43 was also decreased

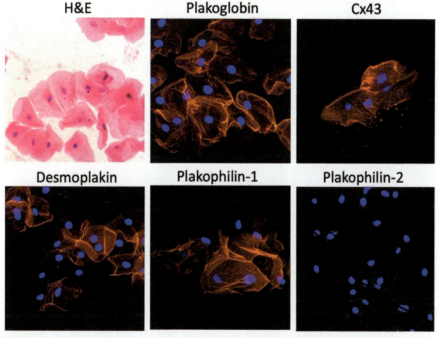

FIGURE 16.6   Representative images of normal buccal mucosa smears. Cells stained with hematoxylin and eosin (H&E) show typical squamous morphology with clearly delineated cell borders. Immunostaining with antibodies against plakoglobin, Cx43, desmoplakin, and plakophilin-1 showed strong immunoreactive signal at the membrane. No specific signal was detected when the cells were immunostained for plakophilin-2; the plakophilin isoform expressed in the heart.[26]

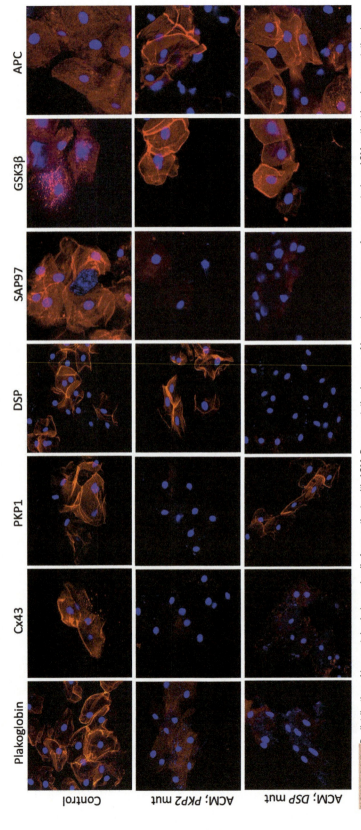

FIGURE 16.7 Redistribution of key proteins in buccal cells from patients with ACM. Representative images of buccal mucosa smears from a control, an ACM patient bearing a mutation in PKP2 and an ACM patient bearing a mutation in *DSP*. Both patients show loss of junctional signal for JUP, Cx43, and SAP97 while in both patients signal for GSK3β and APC is concentrated on the membrane. Only the patient bearing the *PKP2* mutation shows depressed signal for PKP1, while the patient bearing the *DSP* mutation shows depressed signal for DSP.[26]

in the buccal epithelium of a small number of family members examined, who were carriers of pathogenic mutations in desmosomal genes but did not, at the time of analysis, manifest any overt clinical evidence of disease.

Regarding nondesmosomal markers, healthy, control buccal cells show strong junctional signal for SAP97 with diffuse cytosolic localization for GSK3β and APC. In sharp contrast, there is a loss of signal for SAP97 while both GSK3β and APC show a strong signal at the membrane in buccal cells obtained from patients with ACM regardless of the underlying genetic defect (see Figure 16.7).

Although the buccal epithelium consists of terminally differentiated, nondividing cells, if sufficient numbers are obtained, they can be maintained in culture for up to 10 days. Cultured cells from a patient and an unaffected family member bearing a *PKP2* mutation showed loss of immunoreactive signal for Cx43 and a shift of the signal for JUP from the membrane to the cell nuclei. Normal localization for both JUP and Cx43 was restored after the cultured cells were exposed to SB216763 for 24 hours.[26]

Collectively, these results suggest that although the buccal epithelium does not show any overt structural abnormalities in patients diagnosed with ACM, it does show similar patterns of protein distribution changes as those exhibited by cardiac myocytes. Moreover, the fact that buccal mucosa cells can be maintained in culture provides an *ex vivo* model from the patient that could be used to study alterations in signaling pathways and perform drug screens to evaluate potential therapies in patient-specific cells. Much more extensive studies in higher numbers of patients and family members are now required to establish whether buccal mucosa cells can be clinically useful for diagnosis or as a model that will help us uncover mechanisms of disease pathogenesis.

References

1. Thiene G, Basso C. Arrhythmogenic right ventricular cardiomyopathy: An update. *Cardiovasc Pathol.* 2001;10:109–117.

2. Sen-Choedhry S, Syrris P, McKenna WJ. Genetics of right ventricular cardiomyopathy. *J Cardiovasc Electrophysiol.* 2005;16:927–935.

3. Vimalanathan AK, Ehler E, Gehmlich K. Genetics of and pathogenic mechanisms in arrhythmogenic right ventricular cardiomyopathy. *Biophys Rev.* 2018;10:973–982.

4. Zhurinsky J, Shtutman M, Ben-Ze'ev A. Plakoglobin and β-catenin: Protein interactions, regulation and biological roles. *J Cell Sci.* 2000;113:3127–3139.

5. Asimaki A, Saffitz JE. The role of endomyocardial biopsy in ARVC: Looking beyond histology in search of new diagnostic markers. *J Cardiovasc Electrophysiol.* 2011;22:111–117.

6. McKoy G, Protonotarios N, Crosby A, et al. Identification of a deletion in plakoglobin in arrhythmogenic right ventricular cardiomyopathy with palmoplantar keratoderma and woolly hair (Naxos disease). *Lancet.* 2000;355:2119–2124.

7. Kaplan SR, Gard JJ, Protonotarios N, et al. Remodeling of myocyte gap junctions in arrhythmogenic right ventricular cardiomyopathy due to a deletion in plakoglobin (Naxos disease). *Heart Rhythm.* 2004;1:3–11.

8. Norgett EE, Hatsell SJ, Carvajal-Huerta L, et al. Recessive mutation in desmoplakin disrupts desmoplakin-intermediate filament interactions and causes dilated cardiomyopathy, woolly hair and keratoderma. *Hum Mol Genet.* 2000;9:2761–2766.

9. Kaplan SR, Gard JJ, Carvajal-Huerta L, Ruiz-Cabezas JC, Thiene G, Saffitz JE. Structural and molecular pathology of the heart in Carvajal syndrome. *Cardiovasc Pathol.* 2004;12:26–32.

10. Asimaki A, Tandri H, Huang H, et al. A new diagnostic test for arrhythmogenic right ventricular cardiomyopathy. *N Engl J Med.* 2009;360:1075–1084.

11. van der Zwaag PA, van Rijsingen IA, Asimaki A, et al. Phospholamban R14del mutation in patients diagnosed with dilated cardiomyopathy or arrhythmogenic right ventricular cardiomyopathy: Evidence supporting the concept of arrhythmogenic cardiomyopathy. *Eur J Heart Fail.* 2012;14:1199–1207.

12. Saffitz JE. Dependence of electrical coupling on mechanical coupling in cardiac myocytes. In: Thiene G, Pessina AC, editors. *Advances in Cardiovascular Medicine.* Universita degli Studi di Padova, 2003;15–28.

13. Sato PY, Musa H, Coombs W, et al. Loss of plakophilin-2 expression leads to decreased sodium current and slower conduction velocity in cultured cardiac myocytes. *Circ Res.* 2009;105:523–526.

14. Cerrone M, Noorman M, Lin X, et al. Sodium current deficit and arrhythmogenesis in a murine model of plakophilin-2 haploinsufficiency. *Cardiovasc Res.* 2012;95:460–468.

15. Delmar M. The intercalated disk as a single functional unit. *Heart Rhythm.* 2004;1:12–13.

16. Noorman M, Hakim S, Kessler E, et al. Remodeling of the cardiac sodium channel, connexin43, and plakoglobin at the intercalated disk in patients with arrhythmogenic cardiomyopathy. *Heart Rhythm.* 2013;10:412–419.

17. Asimaki A, Kapoor S, Plovie E, et al. Identification of a new modulator of the intercalated disc in a zebrafish model of arrhythmogenic cardiomyopathy. *Sci Transl Med.* 2014;6:240ra74.

18. Cerrone M, Lin X, Zhang M, et al. Missense mutations in plakophilin-2 cause sodium current deficit and associate with a Brugada syndrome phenotype. *Circulation.* 2014;129:1092–1103.

19. Kim C, Wong J, Wen J, et al. Studying arrhythmogenic right ventricular dysplasia with patient-specific iPSCs. *Nature.* 2013; 494:105–110.

20. Milstein ML, Musa H, Balbuena DP, et al. Dynamic reciprocity of sodium and potassium channel expression in a macromolecular complex controls cardiac excitability and arrhythmia. *Proc Natl Acad Sci USA.* 2012;109:E2134–2143.

21. Chelko SP, Asimaki A, Andersen P, et al. Central role for GSK3β in the pathogenesis of arrhythmogenic cardiomyopathy. *JCI Insight.* 2016;1:pii 85923.

22. Chelko SP, Asimaki A, Lowenthal J, et al. Therapeutic modulation of the immune response in arrhythmogenic cardiomyopathy. *Circulation.* 2019;140(18):1491–1505. doi.org/10.1161/CIRCULATIONAHA .119.040676

23. Sugden PH, Fuller SJ, Weiss SC, Clerk A. Glycogen synthase kinase 3 (GSK3) in the heart: A point of integration in hypertrophic signalling and a therapeutic target? A critical analysis. *Br J Pharmacol.* 2008;153(Suppl 1):S137–S153.

24. Swope D, Li J, Radice GL. Beyond cell adhesion: The role of armadillo proteins in the heart. *Cell Signal.* 2013;25:93–100.

25. Caspi O, Huber I, Gepstein A, Arbel G, Maizels L, Boulos M, Gepsein L. Modeling of arrhythmogenic right ventricular cardiomyopathy with human induced pluripotent stem cells. *Circ Cardiovasc Genet.* 2013;6:557–568.

26. Asimaki A, Protonotarios A, James CA, et al. Characterizing the molecular pathology of arrhythmogenic cardiomyopathy in patient buccal mucosa cells. *Circ Arrhythm Electrophysiol.* 2016;9(2):e003688.

27. Hartzfeld M. Plakophilins: Multifunctional proteins or just regulators of desmosomal adhesion? *Biochim Biophys Acta.* 2007;1773:69–77.

28. Neuber S, Mühmer M, Wratten D, Koch PJ, Moll R, Schmidt A. The desmosomal plaque proteins of the plakophilin family. *Dermatol Res Pract.* 2010;2010:101452.

17

The Zurich ARVC Program

Deniz Akdis, MD; Ardan M. Saguner, MD; Corinna Brunckhorst, MD; Firat Duru, MD

Introduction

Although the first cases of right ventricular (RV) dysfunction had been reported in the first half of the 18th century by Giovanni Maria Lancisii, an Italian anatomist and epidemiologist, who reported on 4 generations in a family with dilatation and aneurysms of the RV and sudden death,[1] the disease arrhythmogenic right ventricular cardiomyopathy (ARVC) itself was first described over 200 years later in 1982 by Dr. Frank Marcus and Dr. Guy Fontaine. These pioneers described the disease as *RV dysplasia* in 24 patients.[2] They first characterized some fundamental clinical elements of the disease, such as electrocardiogram (ECG) abnormalities as well as transthoracic echocardiographic (TTE) features of an enlarged aneurysmal RV with a normal left ventricle (LV).

In 1986, in the Greek island of Naxos, Dr. Nikos Protonotarios and Dr. Adalena Tsatsopoulou reported 9 patients with an enlarged RV and palmoplantar keratosis, of whom 7 had a heart disease and one patient died suddenly.[3] The disease, which was named *Naxos disease*, represents an autosomal recessive form of ARVC. The first pathological correlations with the typical clinical picture of ARVC, also associated with sudden death, were described in Italy, particularly after the publication of the original Task Force Criteria (TFC) in 1994.[4] The need to establish large national registries to acquire further knowledge and competence grew even more. Working groups in Italy, Germany, and the Netherlands started establishing national registries to increase the size of the cohorts, including patients and also relatives to gain more information about this heterogeneous cardiomyopathy with highly variable expression.[5,6] In North America, a large ARVC registry was established in the 1980s at Johns Hopkins Hospital in Baltimore.[7-10] In 2001, the Study Group on arrhythmogenic right ventricular dysplasia/cardiomyopathy (ARVD/C) of the Working Groups on Myocardial and Pericardial

Disease and Arrhythmias of the European Society of Cardiology was established and coordinated from Padua,[11] and at the same time "The Multidisciplinary Study of Right Ventricular Dysplasia Investigators in North America" was coordinated by Dr. Frank Marcus.[12] The comprehensive research of these large registries set the ground for the 2010 revised ARVC TFC for the diagnosis of ARVC.[13]

Together with a multidisciplinary team, Professors Duru and Brunckhorst have also been treating ARVC patients in Switzerland since the early 2000s and gained experience in this field. They recognized that due to the geographical location of Switzerland providing a great ethnical diversity, proximity to northern Italy, and the fact that its population is generally physically very active, it may hold a special position in the ARVC research field. Therefore, for many years they saw the need for a national ARVC registry. In 2011, thanks to the support of one of the largest Swiss private foundations, the Bertha and Georg Schwyzer-Winiker Foundation, the Zurich ARVC Program was founded at the University Hospital Zurich. It serves as a national and international center of excellence, which aims to improve the understanding of ARVC and to provide expert care for patients with this complex disease, with state-of-the-art imaging, device therapy, catheter ablation, genetic testing, and genetic counseling, as well as educational platforms, workshops, and events for patients and family members. Since the publication of the first edition of "Current Concepts in Arrhythmogenic RV Cardiomyopathy/Dysplasia" in 2014, the Zurich ARVC Program expanded through various research projects and collaborations focusing on early diagnosis, risk stratification, and prognostic factors.

ARVC Registry and Biobank

The Zurich ARVC Program started enrolling patients in 2011, after ethical approval was obtained. Since then, suspected ARVC cases

referred to the Zurich University Heart Center are evaluated by an interdisciplinary team of electrophysiologists, heart failure specialists, imaging specialists, and cardiac genetic specialists. Furthermore, close collaboration with cardiac pathologists and the Forensic Institute of the University of Zurich enable a better understanding of sudden death cases. Moreover, members of the Zurich ARVC Program regularly visit participating study sites to collect/manage patient data. University hospitals in Bern, Basel, Lausanne, Geneva, and Lugano as well as most state and private hospitals across the country collaborate in this registry. In recent years, there has also been extensive collaboration with centers from other European countries, North America, and China.

Acquisition and analysis of data regarding clinical presentation, longitudinal follow-up, and outcomes of ARVC index patients and family members remain a key element of the Zurich ARVC Program. The electronic registry, based on a secure web-based platform, is regularly updated in each clinical visit. Apart from classical ARVC, the Zurich ARVC Program also focuses on subgroups of patients with different genetic backgrounds and its phenocopies of the disease.

The tissue and blood biobank, which is one of the largest in the field, has extended over the years. Blood samples for DNA and biomarker analysis are being obtained from index patients and family members. Furthermore, the biobank also contains plasma and serum samples as well as endomyocardial and skin biopsies. Using skin biopsies and blood, the team collaborates with other research institutes to obtain patient-specific induced pluripotent stem cell-derived cardiomyocytes (iPSC-CMs) to study epigenetic changes and therapeutic targets. Furthermore, tissue and plasma transcriptome and proteome analyses are performed to obtain disease-specific profiles and identify key molecules that may serve as diagnostic and prognostic biomarkers, and targets for therapeutic interventions (**Figure 17.1**).

Research Projects

The Zurich ARVC Program has focused on following research missions and goals: genotype–phenotype correlations and updating genetic evidence, identification of novel genes, early diagnosis and diagnostic validation, development of prognostic parameters and risk stratification, epigenetic factors, biomarkers, and evaluating patient-specific therapy options with a special attention to translational bench-to-bedside approaches.

Clinical Research

Diagnostic Validation and Risk Stratification

With data from the Zurich ARVC clinical registry, the focus has been on the validation and evolution of the 2010 revised TFC for diagnosis of ARVC, since disease detection of less severe forms, as well as differentiation from phenocopies such as cardiac sarcoidosis or the athlete's heart with similar clinical presentations, remains challenging.

To validate the imaging criteria from the 2010 TFC, the team focused on RV outflow tract (RVOT) dilatation and compared measurements of end-diastolic RVOT diameters between TTE and cardiac magnetic resonance (CMR) imaging, and demonstrated that an additional RVOT diameter defined by the parasternal long-axis M-mode provided the best agreement between the 2 imaging modalities.[14]

A more recent study has identified clinical variables to more accurately discriminate between patients with genetically determined ARVC and cardiac sarcoidosis, in cases fulfilling the definite ARVC 2010 TFC. It was observed that sarcoidosis patients presented with longer PR intervals, advanced atrioventricular block, longer QRS duration, and positive cardiac[18] F-fluorodeoxyglucose PET ([18]FDG-PET) scans. This study also highlighted the role of novel hybrid imaging techniques in improving diagnosis of ARVC (**Figure 17.2**).[15]

Several other clinical parameters and established biomarkers and their effects on long-term clinical outcome were also evaluated. The impact of exercise on biventricular involvement was evaluated. Moreover, plasma high-sensitivity troponin and N-terminal pro-brain natriuretic peptide (NT-proBNP) at baseline were associated with biventricular involvement at later disease stages.[16] In another study, potential thromboembolic complications such as ventricular thrombus formation, which can occur in both ventricles, was characterized (**Figure 17.3**).[17]

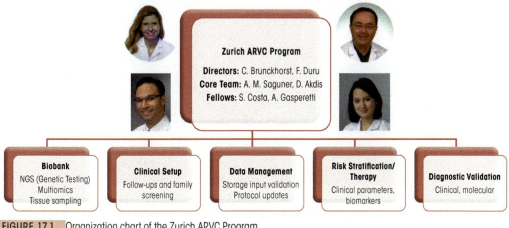

Zurich ARVC Program

Directors: C. Brunckhorst, F. Duru
Core Team: A. M. Saguner, D. Akdis
Fellows: S. Costa, A. Gasperetti

Biobank
NGS (Genetic Testing)
Multiomics
Tissue sampling

Clinical Setup
Follow-ups and family screening

Data Management
Storage input validation
Protocol updates

Risk Stratification/ Therapy
Clinical parameters, biomarkers

Diagnostic Validation
Clinical, molecular

FIGURE 17.1 Organization chart of the Zurich ARVC Program.

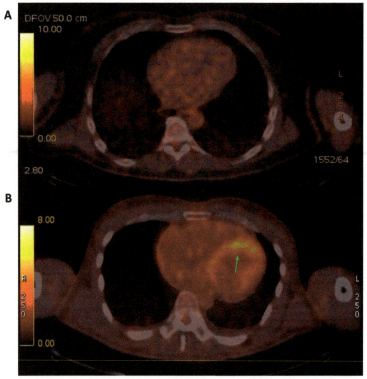

FIGURE 17.2 Differentiating cardiac sarcoidosis from ARVC is presented. **Upper Panel:** [18]FDG-PET of an ARVC patient shows no hypermetabolic activity of myocardium. **Lower Panel:** [18]FDG-PET of a cardiac sarcoidosis patient shows areas of hypermetabolic activity in the septal and anterior area of the LV (**arrow**). (Gasperetti et al., *Heart Rhythm*. 2020;S1547-5271(20)30897-3.[15])

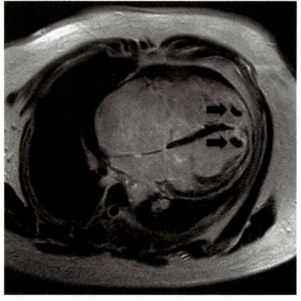

FIGURE 17.3 Thrombus formation in ARVC. Biventricular thrombi in a patient with ARVC and biventricular involvement, detected by CMR (4-chamber view). Thrombus is indicated with **black arrows**.[17] (Figure from Akdis et al., *Thromb Haemost*. 2019;119(8):1373–1378.[17])

For risk stratification in ARVC, the role of electrophysiology (EP) study was investigated in a study, in which inducibility of sustained monomorphic ventricular tachycardia (VT) was shown to be associated with unfavorable outcomes.[18] To investigate the value of ECG findings in predicting adverse outcomes in ARVC, ECGs of 111 patients were screened, which showed that T-wave inversions in inferior leads and a precordial QRS amplitude ratio of ≤ 0.48, as well as QRS fragmentation, constitute valuable variables to predict adverse outcomes.[19] The novel 16-lead high-definition ECG (Schiller, Switzerland) was shown to be beneficial in yielding QRS fragmentation.[20] The value of standard 2-dimensional TTE in the prediction of adverse events was investigated in another study, which showed that fractional area change, tricuspid annulus plane systolic excursion, and RV dilatation were associated with an increased risk of adverse events.[21] Recently, a global multicenter study introduced a risk calculator to estimate the individual risk for sustained ventricular and life-threatening ventricular arrhythmias (VAs). Seven risk factors were identified: age, gender, syncope in the last 6 months, nonsustained VT, and number of ECG leads with T-wave inversions. This calculator can be integrated into daily clinical work to help in the decision process for implantable cardioverter-defibrillator (ICD) implantation (www.arvcrisk.com).[22]

Evaluation of the Current Diagnostic Criteria and Differential Diagnosis

In 2019, an international expert report was published that recognized the pitfalls of the 2010 TFC and highlighted potential limitations of the current criteria and proposed improvements. The following key points were highlighted in this important consensus paper: (1) limitations in the current understanding of the genetic background; (2) the improvement of interpretation of tissue by CMR; (3) the broad spectrum of ARVC phenotypes including left-dominant disease variants; and (4) the special clinical features and diagnostic tests for ARVC in the pediatric population.[23]

Genetic Variants of ARVC

Since the influence of the genetic background on phenotypic manifestation in ARVC remains incompletely understood, genotype-phenotype correlations were studied using next-generation sequencing (NGS). Since 2014, NGS is routinely offered to all index ARVC patients from our registry, and over 100 cardiomyopathy genes are being sequenced. In a study using whole exome sequencing (WES) in ARVC patients and later focusing on 96 cardiomyopathy, and channelopathy-associated genes, we showed that patients with a definite ARVC diagnosis more often presented with pathogenic variants and that patients with a possible diagnosis more often presented with rare variants in other cardiomyopathy-associated genes. This study highlighted the importance of NGS using larger panels including cardiomyopathy-associated genes to differentiate between ARVC and its overlapping phenotypes.

In the Zurich ARVC cohort, around 50% of patients with a definite ARVC diagnosis harbor a desmosomal variant, with plakophilin-2 and desmoglein-2 variants being the most common, whereas around 30% of patients are gene elusive. A small number of patients also present with nondesmosomal variants, but little is known about the disease course in those cases. We studied clinical and imaging data of 65 patients, and showed that patients with multiple and nondesmosomal variants initially presented with normal LV function, and later developed LV dysfunction.[16] Similar data were obtained in a collaborative study with the Fuwai Hospital in Beijing, China, where the influence of variants on outcome was studied in 186 patients and showed that patients with plakophillin-2 variants more often developed VAs, whereas patients with desmoplakin variants and nondesmosomal variants developed biventricular heart failure (unpublished data).

A difficult and widely discussed aspect of genetic testing is the interpretation of genetic variants. Therefore, we focused on genetic reclassification according to the 2015 American College of Medical Genetics (ACMG) criteria in 79 patients. Approximately half of genetic variants were reclassified, with nine patients losing their definite disease status. This study highlighted the utmost importance of periodic state-of-the-art reassessment of genetic variants for an appropriate management of index patients and family members (Costa S. et al. *Circulation: Genomics and Precision Medicine*. 2020. In Press).[24]

Translational Research

Molecular Mechanisms of ARVC

To understand the pathways that play a role in the pathogenesis of ARVC, the Zurich ARVC Program focuses on transcriptomic and proteomic analyses, investigating the expression of mRNA and proteins in tissue and plasma of ARVC patients. This can enable the identification of pathogenic pathways and key upregulated molecules that can serve as biomarkers enabling early diagnosis and prognostic predictions. Initially, we analyzed 60 mRNA molecules in myocardial tissue of 10 ARVC patients and compared this to myocardial tissue of patients with dilated cardiomyopathy and healthy controls. We demonstrated that certain molecules involved in the expression profiles of sarcolemmal calcium channel regulation, apoptosis, and adipogenesis were upregulated in ARVC patients.[25] In a next step, we analyzed over 25'000 mRNA molecules and more than 6'000 proteins in heart tissue. Focusing on adipogenetic/inflamma-

tory and calcium channel regulating pathways, we were able to identify key molecules upregulated specifically in myocardium of ARVC patients. In a further step, these biomarkers are being validated to evaluate their clinical use.[26]

In order to assess the role of sex hormones, we collaborated with Professor V. Chen's group (Indiana, USA) who first studied ARVC in patient-derived induced pluripotent stem cells (iPSCs).[27] Since male patients tend to develop the disease earlier and often present with more severe phenotypes as compared to women, we hypothesized that serum levels of sex hormones could contribute to major arrhythmic cardiovascular events in ARVC. We were able to demonstrate that in male patients suffering from major arrhythmic events, testosterone levels were significantly higher, whereas in females with arrhythmic events, estradiol levels were lower. We tested the potential mechanisms on patient-specific iPSC models and demonstrated that testosterone worsened and estradiol improved cardiomyocyte apoptosis and lipogenesis. These findings support a potential role of sex hormones in the pathophysiology of ARVC (**Figure 17.4**).[28]

Biomarkers in ARVC for Risk Assessment and Therapeutic Indications

Another intense collaboration was with the ARVC research group of Professor R. Hamilton at the Hospital for Sick Children & Research Institute, University of Toronto, Canada, focusing on autoimmune processes in ARVC and its phenocopies. Western blot and enzyme-linked immunosorbent assay (ELISA) identified anti-desmoglein-2 autoantibodies in serum of ARVC patients that were upregulated and correlated with disease severity. For the first time, this study showed that next to genetic variants, autoimmune mecha-

Cardiomyocyte apoptosis and lipogenesis

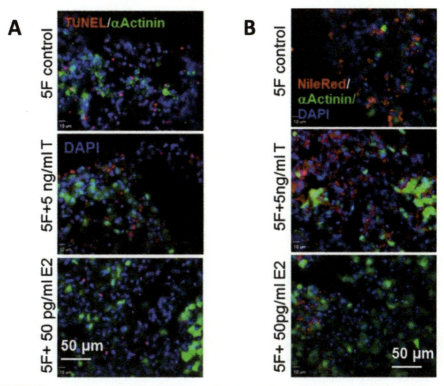

FIGURE 17.4   Influence of sex hormones on ARVC iPSC-CMs. **Panel A:** Testosterone (T) increased and estradiol (E2) decreased CM apoptosis (TUNEL staining in **red,** DAPI = nucleus). **Panel B:** CM lipid accumulation is increased by testosterone (T) and decreased by estradiol (E2); lipid accumulation = Nile Red-positive lipid droplets. (Representative images of 2-week 5F-treated JK#11 ARVC/D iPSC-CMs.) (Figure from Akdis et al., *Eur Heart J.* 2017;38(19):1498–1508.[28])

nisms may also play an important role in this disease.[29] We currently assess the specificity of this biomarker in phenocopies of ARVC such as cardiac sarcoidosis (unpublished data).

The prediction of the course of disease in ARVC, especially with respect to biventricular involvement, remains challenging. There are no validated prognostic biomarkers for biventricular involvement and heart failure in ARVC. Together with the research group from the Fuwai Hospital, we investigated the circulating levels of sST2, GDF-15, and plasma NT-proBNP, and showed that the combination of these 3 biomarkers may best predict biventricular involvement in ARVC (unpublished data) (**Figure 17.5**).

Studying Hemodynamic Changes in an In Vitro Right Heart Model

The mechanisms that lead to RV dysfunction remain incompletely understood. Therefore, together with the Institute of Hydromechanics at the Swiss Federal Institute of Technology (ETH), Switzerland, we studied hemodynamic changes that may lead to RV dysfunction. For this purpose, a novel and anatomically accurate compliant silicone right heart model derived from a high-resolution CMR scan of a healthy male control was developed and 3D Particle Tracking Velocimetry (3D-PTV), a novel optical imaging method, was used. RV and RVOT flow patterns at resting conditions were

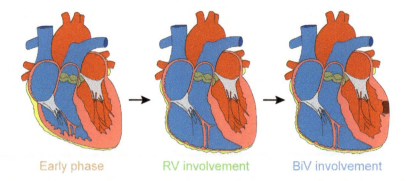

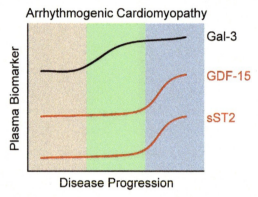

FIGURE 17.5   Fibrosis biomarkers and disease progression. Plasma levels of sST2, GDF-15, and Gal-3 are elevated in ARVC patients with biventricular involvement, and hence, these biomarkers are correlated with adverse heart failure outcomes, whereas Gal-3 may be an isolated biomarker for fibrosis (unpublished data).

obtained from healthy controls and ARVC patients using phase-contrast CMR, and our findings from the in vitro model were validated *in vivo*. Our results showed that in healthy and diseased hearts, there was an increase in wall shear stress in the RVOT relative to the rest of the RV. Higher peak wall shear stress magnitudes were found for the diseased cases. Our results help to explain why the RVOT is frequently involved in ARVC, and why continuation of exercise may lead to adverse remodeling at this predilection site (**Figure 17.6**).[30]

Zurich International Symposium on Arrhythmogenic Cardiomyopathies

Since the first international ARVC symposium was held in 2012 in Zurich, Switzerland, the meeting has grown, becoming a tradition and one of the most important international meetings on this topic. In September 2019, the conference was held for a fourth time, for three days, focusing on clinical updates and basic and translational research. Moreover, in the setting of this symposium, the Zurich ARVC Research Prizes were awarded for the third time to scientists who published the best research studies in basic and clinical sciences in the field of ARVC.

Conclusions

Since the first edition of this book, the Zurich ARVC Program has contributed significantly, with multiple basic and clinical studies, to the understanding of ARVC. We are truly indebted to our national and international colleagues for the close collaboration. In the coming years, our program will continue to

A

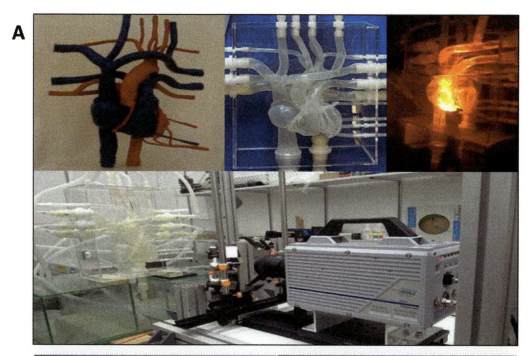

B

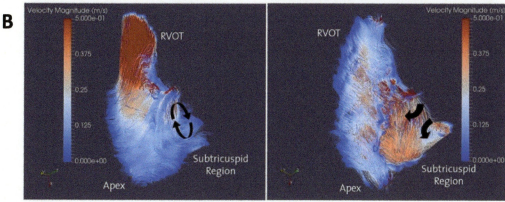

FIGURE 17.6 Investigation of flow patterns and mechanical stresses in the RV using a novel heart model.
Panel A: Workflow for the assessment of velocity information in the right heart model. Model was created using a high-resolution CMR heart scan of a healthy male. Silicone model cast was 3D printed accordingly. 3D particle tracking velocimetry measurements have been performed in the anatomically accurate right heart model. Streamlines color-coded with velocity magnitude were obtained along the superior vena cava, inferior vena cava, right atrium, RV, and RVOT.
Panel B: Streamlines color-coded with velocity magnitude were obtained along the RV at peak systolic phase (**left**) and mid-diastolic phase (**right**) obtained by using MR dimensions of a healthy athletic male. **Red** color is for high velocity; **blue color** is for slow velocity. **Arrow** indicates recirculation regions at ventricular filling. (Figure from Gülan et al., *Sci Rep.* 2019;9(1):100.[30])

have the same main focus—creating awareness for and broadening knowledge on this challenging disease.

Acknowledgments

The Zurich ARVC Program is supported by research grants from the Bertha and Georg Schwyzer-Winiker Foundation, Baugarten Foundation, Dr. Hans-Peter Wild / USZ Foundation, Swiss Heart Foundation and Swiss National Science Foundation.

References

1. Lancisii JM. *De motu cordis et aneurysmatibus opus postumum in duas partes divisum*, 1738.

2. Marcus FI, Fontaine GH, Guiraudon G, et al. Right ventricular dysplasia: A report of 24 adult cases. *Circulation*. 1982;65(2):384–398.

3. Protonotarios N, Tsatsopoulou A, Patsourakos P, et al. Cardiac abnormalities in familial palmoplantar keratosis. *Br Heart J*. 1986;56(4):321–326.

4. McKenna WJ, Thiene G, Nava A, et al. Diagnosis of arrhythmogenic right ventricular dysplasia/cardiomyopathy: Task Force of the Working Group Myocardial and Pericardial Disease of the European Society of Cardiology and of the Scientific Council on Cardiomyopathies of the International Society and Federation of Cardiology. *Br Heart J*. 1994;71(3):215–218.

5. Basso C, Corrado D, Thiene G. Cardiovascular causes of sudden death in young individuals including athletes. *Cardiol Rev*. 1999;7(3):127–135.

6. Corrado D, Thiene G, Nava A, Rossi L, Pennelli N. Sudden death in young competitive athletes: Clinicopathologic correlations in 22 cases. *Am J Med*. 1990;89(5):588–596.

7. Nasir K, Bomma C, Tandri H, et al. Electrocardiographic features of arrhythmogenic right ventricular dysplasia/cardiomyopathy according to disease severity: A need to broaden diagnostic criteria. *Circulation*. 2004;110(12):1527–1534.

8. Bhonsale A, Groeneweg JA, James CA, et al. Impact of genotype on clinical course in arrhythmogenic right ventricular dysplasia/cardiomyopathy-associated mutation carriers. *Eur Heart J*. 2015;36(14):847–855.

9. Dalal D, Jain R, Tandri H, et al. Long-term efficacy of catheter ablation of ventricular tachycardia in patients with arrhythmogenic right ventricular dysplasia/cardiomyopathy. *J Am Coll Cardiol*. 2007;50(5):432–440.

10. Ruwald AC, Marcus F, Estes NA, et al. Association of competitive and recreational sport participation with cardiac events in patients with arrhythmogenic right ventricular cardiomyopathy: Results from the North American multidisciplinary study of arrhythmogenic right ventricular cardiomyopathy. *Eur Heart J*. 2015;36(27):1735–1743.

11. Basso C, Wichter T, Danieli GA, et al. Arrhythmogenic right ventricular cardiomyopathy: Clinical registry and database, evaluation of therapies, pathology registry, DNA banking. *Eur Heart J*. 2004;25(6):531–534.

12. Marcus F, Towbin JA, Zareba W, et al. Arrhythmogenic right ventricular dysplasia/cardiomyopathy (ARVD/C): A multidisciplinary study: Design and protocol. *Circulation*. 2003;107(23):2975–2978.

13. Marcus FI, McKenna WJ, Sherrill D, et al. Diagnosis of arrhythmogenic right ventricular cardiomyopathy/dysplasia: Proposed modification of the Task Force Criteria. *Eur Heart J*. 2010;31(7):806–814.

14. Saguner AM, Gotschy A, Niemann M, et al. Right ventricular outflow tract dimensions in arrhythmogenic right ventricular cardiomyopathy/dysplasia: A multicentre study comparing echocardiography and cardiovascular magnetic resonance. *Eur Heart J Cardiovasc Imaging*. 2018;19(5):516–523.

15. Gasperetti A, Rossi V, Chiodini A, et al. Differentiating hereditary arrhythmogenic right ventricular cardiomyopathy from cardiac sarcoidosis fulfilling 2010 ARVC Task Force Criteria. *Heart Rhythm*. 2020;S1547-5271(20)30897-3.

16. Akdis D, Saguner AM, Burri H, et al. Clinical predictors of left ventricular involvement

in arrhythmogenic right ventricular cardiomyopathy. *Am Heart J.* 2020;223:34–43.

17. Akdis D, Chen K, Saguner AM, et al. Clinical characteristics of patients with a right ventricular thrombus in arrhythmogenic right ventricular cardiomyopathy. *Thromb Haemost.* 2019;119(8):1373–1378.

18. Saguner AM, Medeiros-Domingo A, Schwyzer MA, et al. Usefulness of inducible ventricular tachycardia to predict long-term adverse outcomes in arrhythmogenic right ventricular cardiomyopathy. *Am J Cardiol.* 2013;111(2):250–257.

19. Saguner AM, Ganahl S, Baldinger SH, et al. Usefulness of electrocardiographic parameters for risk prediction in arrhythmogenic right ventricular dysplasia. *Am J Cardiol.* 2014;113(10):1728–1734.

20. Li GL, Saguner AM, Akdis D, Fontaine GH. Value of a novel 16-lead high-definition ECG machine to detect conduction abnormalities in structural heart disease. *Pacing Clin Electrophysiol.* 2018;41(6):643–655.

21. Saguner AM, Vecchiati A, Baldinger SH, et al. Different prognostic value of functional right ventricular parameters in arrhythmogenic right ventricular cardiomyopathy/dysplasia. *Circ Cardiovasc Imaging.* 2014;7(2):230–239.

22. Cadrin-Tourigny J, Bosman LP, Nozza A, et al. A new prediction model for ventricular arrhythmias in arrhythmogenic right ventricular cardiomyopathy. *Eur Heart J.* 2019;40(23):1850–1858.

23. Corrado D, van Tintelen PJ, McKenna WJ, et al. Arrhythmogenic right ventricular cardiomyopathy: Evaluation of the current diagnostic criteria and differential diagnosis. *Eur Heart J.* 2020;41(14):1414–1429.

24. Costa S. et al. Impact of genetic variant reassessment on the diagnosis of arrhythmogenic right ventricular cardiomyopathy Based on the 2010 Task Force Criteria. *Circulation: Genomics and Precision Medicine.* 2020. In Press.

25. Akdis D, Medeiros-Domingo A, Gaertner-Rommel A, et al. Myocardial expression profiles of candidate molecules in arrhythmogenic right ventricular cardiomyopathy/dysplasia compared with dilated cardiomyopathy and healthy controls. *Heart Rhythm.* 2016 Mar;13(3):731–741.

26. Akdis D, Saguner A, Matter C, et al. Identification of novel biomarkers for diagnosis of arrhythmogenic right ventricular cardiomyopathy using transcriptomics and label-free proteomics. *Eur Heart J.* ESC Congress 2018; 1036.

27. Kim C, Wong J, Wen J, et al. Studying arrhythmogenic right ventricular dysplasia with patient-specific iPSCs. *Nature.* 2013;494(7435):105–110.

28. Akdis D, Saguner AM, Shah K, et al. Sex hormones affect outcome in arrhythmogenic right ventricular cardiomyopathy/dysplasia: From a stem cell derived cardiomyocyte-based model to clinical biomarkers of disease outcome. *Eur Heart J.* 2017;38(19):1498–1508.

29. Chatterjee D, Fatah M, Akdis D, et al. An autoantibody identifies arrhythmogenic right ventricular cardiomyopathy and participates in its pathogenesis. *Eur Heart J.* 2018;39(44):3932–3944.

30. Gülan U, Saguner AM, Akdis D, et al. Hemodynamic changes in the right ventricle induced by variations of cardiac output: A possible mechanism for arrhythmia occurrence in the outflow tract. *Sci Rep.* 2019;9(1):100.

Impressions from the
Zurich International Symposium on
Arrhythmogenic Cardiomyopathies
2019

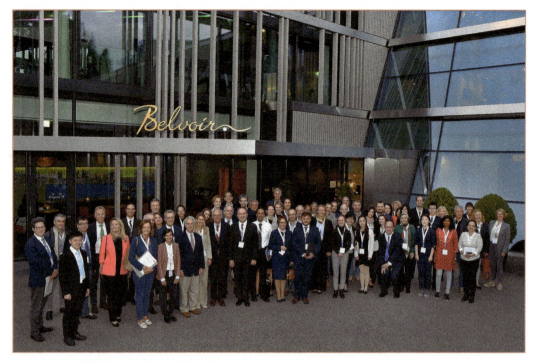

GROUP PHOTO AT ZURICH INTERNATIONAL SYMPOSIUM ON ARRHYTHMOGENIC CARDIOMYOPATHIES, HELD ON 26-28 SEPTEMBER 2019 IN RÜSCHLIKON, SWITZERLAND.

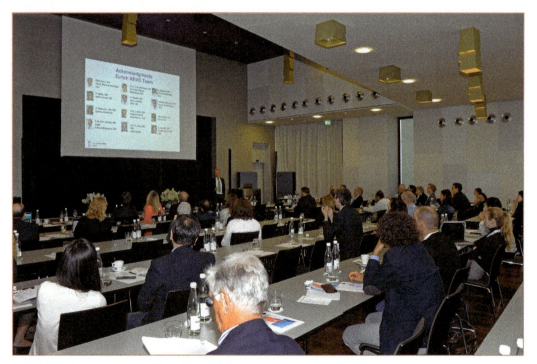

ATTENDEES OF THE SYMPOSIUM LISTENING TO THE PRESENTATION OF FRANK RUSCHITZKA.

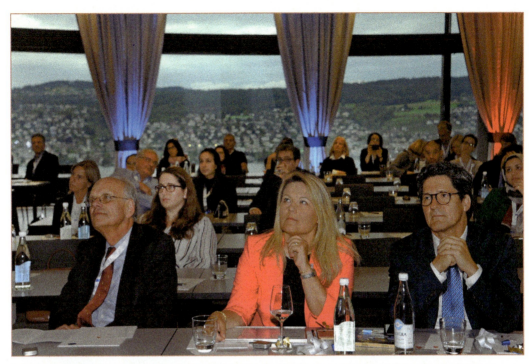

FACULTY MEMBERS OF THE SYMPOSIUM IN THE CONFERENCE ROOM. FIRST ROW (L) TO (R): RICHARD HAUER, MARINA CERRONE, MARIO DELMAR.

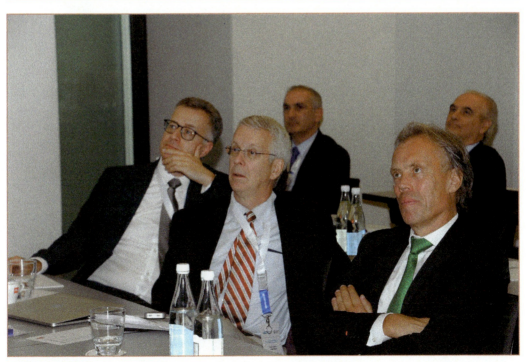

FACULTY MEMBERS OF THE SYMPOSIUM IN THE CONFERENCE ROOM. (L) TO (R): PERRY ELLIOTT, HUGH CALKINS, CHRISTOPHER SEMSARIAN, FRANK RUSCHITZKA, DOMENICO CORRADO.

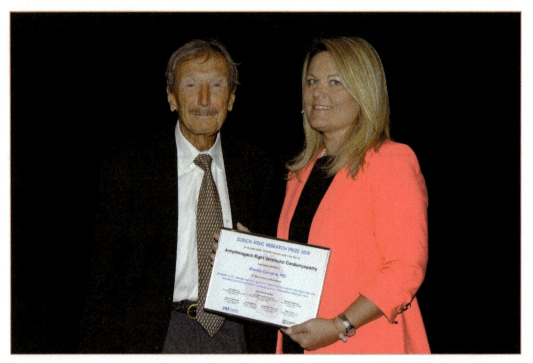

MARINA CERRONE RECEIVING THE 2019 ZURICH ARVC BASIC SCIENCE RESEARCH PRIZE FROM ROLF M. ZINKERNAGEL, 1996 NOBEL PRIZE LAUREATE IN PHYSIOLOGY AND MEDICINE.

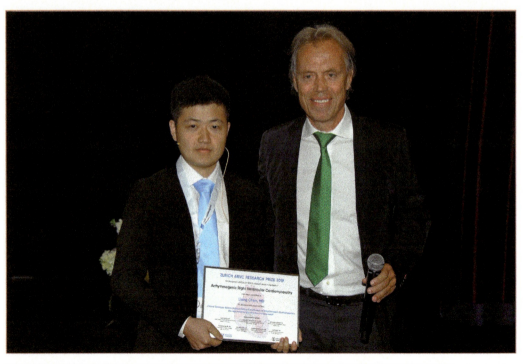

LIANG CHEN RECEIVING THE 2019 ZURICH ARVC CLINICAL SCIENCE RESEARCH PRIZE FROM FRANK RUSCHITZKA, CHAIRMAN OF CARDIOLOGY AT THE UNIVERSITY HEART CENTER ZURICH.

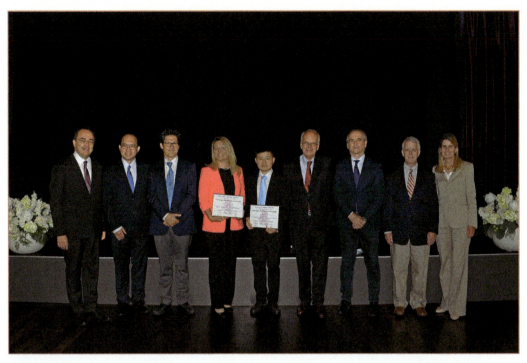

ZURICH ARVC RESEARCH PRIZE COMMITTEE AND AWARDEES: (L) TO (R): FIRAT DURU, VINCENT CHEN, MARIO DELMAR, MARINA CERRONE, LIANG CHEN, RICHARD HAUER, DOMENICO CORRADO, HUGH CALKINS, CORINNA BRUNCKHORST.

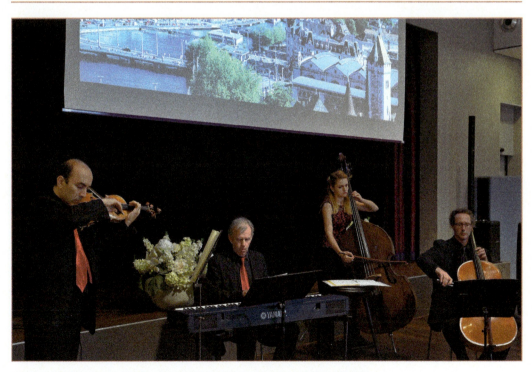

MUSICAL OPENING OF THE ZURICH ARVC RESEARCH PRIZE CEREMONY (MUSICI VOLANTI).

Index

Page numbers followed by f and t refer to figures and tables, respectively.